Health Care
Law and Ethics

Health Care
Law and Ethics

American Association of Medical Assistants
Chicago

Health Care Law and Ethics

Published by the
American Association of Medical Assistants, Inc.
20 North Wacker Drive, Suite 1575
Chicago, Illinois 60606-2903

This is a revised edition of *Law for the Medical Office*, a book
previously published by the American Association of Medical
Assistants, Inc.

ISBN Number: 0-942732-02-2

Table of Contents

List of Figures

Foreword

It is no longer true that a physician can practice his/her profession essentially alone. Why is this so?

A number of events have transpired in medicine during the past few years. There have been tremendous advances in the science of medicine, with a concomitant proliferation of medical and allied health personnel to help meet the demands of those advances. Social values have changed, necessitating a change in the art of practicing medicine, particularly in the areas of patients' rights involving privacy and confidentiality, informed consent, access to medical records, and the right to refuse treatment. There has been an almost unbelievable change in our ethical and moral standards surrounding the delivery of medical care—e.g., contraception, sterilization, abortion, and in vitro and in vivo fertilization.

Commensurate with all these changes, there is also the increased ability of the physician to relieve pain, cure disease, replace parts, and prolong life. The healer now has the ability to sustain "life" when it no longer has any meaningful quality, as in "brain death."

The paperwork involved in the practice of medicine today has increased not only because of the complexity of records that must be kept, but also because of the number and sophistication of reimbursement regulations imposed by the government and insurance carriers.

The American Association of Medical Assistants has prepared this text that is easy to read, simple to comprehend, yet highly instructive and educational. The book provides an overview of the law, and is helpful as a reference for dealing with specific problems.

Because it is an overview, however, there is one caveat: The "law" may vary from state to state. It is always prudent and crucial to verify the law in each particular jurisdiction.

Harold L. Hirsch, MD, JD, FCLM, Adjunct Professor
American University,
Catholic University,
George Washington University,
Montgomery College
1984

Foreword to the Revised Edition

In the foreword to the first edition of this book, Dr. Hirsch noted that the physician can no longer practice alone. For a variety of reasons, the increasing shift of responsibility of allied health practitioners has continued. The scope of this revised edition has been expanded to be useful for a greater number of health care and allied health care practitioners. Legal theories and responsibilities related to such problems as invasion of privacy, negligence, and fraud are the same for practitioners in all areas of health care.

When I began using the first edition of this book with my community college students, I was extremely gratified by the outcomes: the students were enthusiastic about the text and workbook; they seemed to understand the concepts with a minimum of difficulty; and they were achieving better grades on examinations and projects. For these reasons, we have endeavored to maintain the "student friendly" aspects in this revised edition.

The straightforward language, the clear explanations of concepts, the frequent competency checks, and the use of cases and examples to clarify concepts that facilitate understanding have all been continued. Chapters such as "Intentional Torts and Criminal Offenses" and "Medical Ethics and Bioethical Issues" have been updated to accommodate more recent advances in science and medicine as well as changes in the law. Two new chapters have been added to address employment and consumer protection laws. As a culmination of the discussion of medical law, we have added a chapter that focuses the reader's attention on avoiding unjustified litigation, especially negligence litigation.

As always, I remind you that it is essential to be knowledgeable about the "law" in your jurisdiction. As Dr. Hirsch noted in 1984, laws do indeed vary from state to state.

Diana Leigh-Hopper, MEd, CMA-A
(formerly Diana Hopper-Bargioni)
West Valley College
Saratoga, California
1996

Acknowledgments

The Continuing Education Board of the American Association of Medical Assistants wishes to acknowledge the extensive research and fine work of the original text's author, Mary Jo Schwartz-Padgett.

We also wish to thank Barbara Ensley, RN, CMA-C, and Mary Lee Seibert, EdD, CMA, for their contributions to the workbook, and the late Rachel K. Younger, CMA-ACP, for her contributions to the medical ethics section of the textbook and answer keys in both text and workbook.

To the staff of the American Medical Association's Office of General Counsel and to Harold L. Hirsch, MD, JD, we express our sincere gratitude for their review of the textbook drafts for medical-legal accuracy.

So many dedicated members of the AAMA contributed their time and efforts to this book that we cannot name all of them here. But one particular group must receive our special thanks: the Task Force to Develop a Course in Medical Law and Ethics, under the leadership of Maedelle Sharpton, MT, CMA-C, Chair.

Acknowledgments to the Revised Edition

The Continuing Education Board gratefully acknowledges the contributions of the individuals who were instrumental in the development and production of this revision:

Diana Leigh-Hopper, MEd, CMA-A, who—as a medical assisting program director with a strong background in law and ethics—is particularly well-suited to serve as revising author for this textbook. The Continuing Education Board is deeply grateful for the time, care, and talent she has devoted to this project.

The manuscript was thoroughly reviewed by Donald A. Balasa, JD, MBA, consulting editor, whose generous sharing of his comprehensive knowledge and involvement with public policy issues affecting the medical assisting profession proved invaluable.

Helpful suggestions for improvement were provided by Loretta M. Hatlestad, CMA, Robin L. Bluestein, CMA-C, and Faith A. Ward, CMA. Their accumulated knowledge and desire for excellence were key elements to the success of this revision.

The cover artwork and design was completed by Anna L. Johnson, with technical assistance provided by Jean M. Lynch.

Much needed additional support was provided by Elliot V. B. Grudem with his legal research and editing contributions, and by Stacey J. Roseen, who provided additional copy and layout editing and prepared the text for print.

Although the Continuing Education Board unfortunately cannot here extend thanks and acknowledgment to every individual who assisted with this project, we proudly highlight the principal contributors to this revised edition.

How to Use This Course

The purpose of this course is to teach allied health professionals about medical law and ethics.

The course includes a textbook which may be used alone or,
as we suggest, in combination with the workbook. You should
also keep a notebook handy to record your responses to the textbook's competency checks and the workbook's essay questions.

Throughout this book actual legal cases illustrating the principles discussed have been summarized and presented. After each
case summary a notation appears identifying the case and indicating where it was first reported and published. Only cases reviewed by appellate courts are published regularly; cases resolved
completely at the trial court level and never appealed generally
are not published. This case identification information is called a
citation. If additional information is desired. the citation gives the
reader enough information to find the complete case report.

Each citation consists of four parts. Case citation *Levy v Kirk,
187 So.2d 401, Fla. 1966* is used to illustrate these parts.

1. The *case name* gives the names of the litigants. In our
    example, someone named Levy sued someone named
    Kirk.
2. The *book* indicates where the case report may be found.
    Books containing case reports are called reporters. Each
    reporter covers a certain geographical area of the country
    and is usually named for that area. Within the citation the
    name of the reporter is usually abbreviated as indicated
    by the following examples of reporters and abbrevia-
    tions: Northeast (NE) Reporter, New York Supplement
    (NYS), Northwest (NW) Reporter, Southern (So)
    Reporter, Southwestern (SW) Reporter, Atlantic (A)
    Reporter, Pacific (P) Reporter. Since each reporter con-
    sists of many, many volumes, the case citation specifies
    the volume number of the reporter, a series number
    (when applicable), and the page number on which the
    case report begins. The book for our case is 187 So.2d
    401; this case is reported in volume 187 of the Southern
    Reporter 2d series, beginning on page 401.

3. The *state* indicates where the case was tried; sometimes, the name of the court is also included in the citation. Our example case was tried in Florida, and the court name was not given.
4. The *year* the decision was made. The decision in *Levy v Kirk* was reached in 1966.

Each chapter of the textbook begins with learning objectives. To help you gauge whether you are understanding the material, competency checks are placed throughout each chapter. We suggest that you stop at each competency check section. In your notebook, write the answers to the questions; try not to refer back to the text. Then, refer to the answer key at the back of the textbook to make certain that your responses were correct. If you responded correctly, continue on to the next section of the chapter. If your responses were not correct, restudy the material before proceeding.

After completing each chapter, turn to the workbook and complete the exercises. When you feel confident that you know the material, take the quiz at the end of the workbook chapter.

Compare your responses to the answer key at the back of the workbook. If you did well, begin the next chapter in your textbook. If you had difficulty, restudy the material and then review the workbook exercises.

The material in the book is cumulative—concepts presented in later chapters build upon information provided earlier. It is very important that you understand each chapter and section before continuing to the next one.

In addition to exercises designed to help you learn the concepts presented in this textbook, the workbook also contains an examination. Five CEU credits may be obtained from the American Association of Medical Assistants for completing the course examination with an average score of 70 percent or better.

Instructions for how to obtain the CEU credit are provided in the workbook. (School copies of the workbook are not eligible for CEU credit.)

Laws vary from state to state, and practices may differ from one community to another, or from one employer to another. This textbook presents the generally acceptable standards. If your employer's policies and procedures seem to differ from examples provided throughout this book, you should confer with your employer to clarify what is expected of you in your specific practice situation.

1

An Introduction to Law

All groups of people have developed rules to live by so that the collective needs of a group cannot be usurped by the wishes of an individual.

Less complex societies than our own have created informal and unwritten rules based on myth, magic, tradition, or religion, which were passed by word of mouth from generation to generation.

More complex societies have evolved formal, written regulations reflecting philosophical, political, and economic values. In this country such regulations are called laws.

Regardless of whether the rules are called traditions or laws, myths or regulations, their function is to govern certain aspects of an individual's behavior and to require adherence to certain behavior.

As a society becomes more complex and impersonal, its members seem increasingly to rely upon laws and the legal system to solve problems and to maintain order.

This is evident in the United States, where the average citizen now calls on the courts to solve problems that were previously accepted and forgotten as a condition of life or mitigated through personal communication or compromise.

Today, many individuals are exercising their constitutional right to bring suit in legal forums ranging from small claims court to the U.S. Supreme Court.

No one has escaped the litigation upsurge, but health care professionals have been prime targets. Self-protection is a primary reason that all health care providers and their employees must be aware of the laws affecting them. More importantly, as practitioners dedicated to the healing arts, health care providers have an even greater obligation to protect the patients from injurious mistakes.

To fulfill this obligation, it is important to understand the legal nature of the doctor-patient relationship. Many of the legal duties—such as the duty to keep patient information confidential—owed a patient by the doctor are also owed by all other caregivers.

Unfortunately, many do not realize that legal considerations affect almost every daily task. It is hoped that the study of the material in this book will increase overall awareness of how the law shapes the professional practice of every health care professional.

This first chapter emphasizes the fundamentals of law and concludes with a brief overview of some medical–legal problems that have arisen during the past twenty years.

OBJECTIVES

After you finish this chapter you will be able to:

1. List four reasons for suits brought against health care professionals today.
2. Distinguish between public and private law.
3. Identify and describe briefly four branches of public law.
4. Identify and describe briefly six branches of private law.
5. Distinguish between the sources of statutory and common law.
6. Distinguish between substantive and procedural law.
7. Describe the three levels of the federal court system.

CONTEMPORARY MEDICAL–LEGAL PROBLEMS

Shortly after World War II, the number of lawsuits against health care providers began to steadily increase and began receiving national attention in the late 1960s.

Causes of Suits

The causes for the increased number of suits against health care providers are many and complex. Some factors contributing to the increase include:

- Scientific advances that enable cures for certain previously untreatable conditions but, at the same time, carry inherent risks of undesirable results or side effects.
- Exaggerated public expectations of what can be accomplished. Many people unrealistically expect a cure for every ailment.
- Reduced communication between physician and patient and the subsequent breakdown of personal rapport. Increased specialization among physicians—a factor related to scientific advancements—has probably contributed a great deal to this breakdown in personal rapport. A poor result—no matter how skillful the treatment—accompanied by a poor doctor–patient relationship, often triggers a lawsuit. According to R. Crawford Morris, an expert defense attorney for physicians, "When the physician–patient rapport remains at a high level of competence and trust, most patients will ride out a bad result through much pain and suffering and expenses, without resort to lawsuit. But when that rapport is inadequate in the beginning, or is permitted to deteriorate en route, a suit is likely to follow."[1]
- An increasingly suit-oriented society that seeks to hold someone at fault for every injury or accident previously attributed to "plain old bad luck."

An increased number of lawsuits against health care providers has had some far-reaching effects.

First, the cost of professional liability insurance has skyrocketed. These costs have been passed on to patients and are one factor contributing to the public outcry over the high cost of medical care.

Second, fearing the possibility of a lawsuit at almost every turn, some health care providers have resorted to practicing "defensive medicine." In some cases, unnecessary tests have been ordered, adding to the cost of care; in other instances, certain desirable tests have not been ordered because of inherent dangers. Whatever the case, it has been contended that the health care provider's fear of a lawsuit has had a detrimental effect on the quality of care provided.

Third, the increased caseload on the judicial system has resulted in long delays between the time a suit is filed and the time it is resolved. Professional negligence suits are unusually complex and lengthy. Add these suits to an already overburdened court system and, too often, the result is a two- to six-year delay between the time a complaint is filed and the final judgment is rendered.

LAW: PUBLIC AND PRIVATE

Laws in the United States are divided into two major categories: public law and private law. Public law defines the rights and responsibilities of government in relation to its citizens and the rights and responsibilities of citizens in relation to their government. Private law, also called civil law, governs certain activities between and among private citizens. Each category can be subdivided into branches of law according to the type of activities and responsibilities involved. (See Figure 1-A, page 7.)

Branches of Public Law

Criminal law defines crimes, describes penalties for offenses, and stipulates procedures for prosecuting offenders. Offenses range from littering to homicide. They include practicing medicine without a license.

Although most crimes occur between or among individuals, criminal acts are so serious and their consequences so dire that the offense is considered an affront to all citizens. The state, therefore, as the representative of its citizens, prosecutes the offender. The victim of the crime may also sue the offender under private law.

Constitutional law defines the rights, responsibilities, and powers of government and citizens. Although the United States Constitution is the foundation of constitutional law, each state has its own constitution describing and stipulating its own rights and powers. Under our form of government, each state has jurisdiction over matters not specifically given the federal government.

Administrative law describes the rights and powers of government agencies. It is the fastest growing branch of law. Agencies are established by the executive branch of government, through order of the legislative branch, and are given the authority to make legally binding rules to carry out their duties. State boards of medical examiners are administrative agencies.

International law deals with treaties, agreements, conflicts, and issues between and among countries such as trade agreements, boundary disputes, and the use of international waters.

Branches of Private Law

Contract law and commercial law concern the rights and obligations of people who enter into contracts. The health care provider-patient relationship represents a contractual agreement governed by the principles of contract law. (See Chapter Three.)

Tort law governs the redress of wrongs or injuries suffered by someone because of another's wrongdoing or misdeed. A tort is a private or civil wrong resulting from the breach of a legal duty. Torts, however, do not encompass breaches of contract. Tort law is the basis of most lawsuits against health care providers. (See Chapter Six.)

Property law governs the ownership of real and personal property.

Inheritance law concerns the transfer of property after the owner's death. It establishes the respective rights of survivors and sets the rules for making wills and trusts.

Family law specifies the rights and obligations of husbands and wives, children and parents. Marriage, divorce, adoption, and child support are the substance of family law.

Corporation law concerns the formation and operation of incorporated businesses. Health care providers who have incorporated are concerned with these laws from a business and tax standpoint. Such matters are not discussed in this book, which is concerned with laws affecting the practice of health care professionals.

Most private or civil law matters are handled out of court. When disputes arise, however, the party who feels wronged may sue the wrongdoer to recover compensation for the alleged wrongdoing. Such disputes are aired in court and decided by a judge or jury according to procedures discussed later in this text.

COMPETENCY CHECK: ONE

1. True or False: Public law governs the responsibilities of government to citizens and of citizens to government.

2. True or False: Private law governs certain activities between and among citizens.

3. True or False: The health care provider-patient relationship is governed in part by principles of contract law.

4. True or False: Tort law is a branch of public law.

5. List at least three factors that have contributed to the increased number of lawsuits against physicians in the past twenty years.

The competency check items should be answered as they appear in the chapters. After recording your answer on a separate sheet of paper, check the accuracy of your responses by referring to the answer key in the Appendix of this book. If you answered correctly, proceed to the next section of this chapter. If you missed one or more questions, restudy the section before proceeding. Follow this procedure throughout the rest of the book.

SOURCES OF LAW

There are two major sources of law: statutory and common.

Statutory Law

Federal and state legislators enact laws known as statutes, which provide the bases of statutory law. (Local governments—county, township, city, for example—may also enact laws pertaining to community or regional matters. Such laws are usually called ordinances.)

Figure 1-A. Branches of Law and Related Subject Matter

PUBLIC LAW

Criminal Law	Constitutional Law	Administrative Law	International Law
Arson	Civil rights	Consumer	Arms control
Bribery	Federal and	protection	Extradition
Burglary	State powers	Environmental	Hijacking
Extortion	Relations	protection	and piracy
Forgery	between states	Interstate	Human rights
Kidnapping	Separation of	commerce	Territorial
Larceny	executive,	Public safety	waters
Manslaughter	judicial and	Social welfare	Uses of outer
Murder	legislative	Taxation	space
Perjury	powers	Workers' wages	Uses of ocean
Rape		and hours	War crimes
Robbery			

PRIVATE LAW

Contract and Commercial Law	Tort Law	Property Law
Credit purchases	Invasion of privacy	Landlord-tenant
Employment contracts	Personal injury	relations
Guarantees	Professional malpractice	Mortgages
Insurance policies	Slander and libel	Transfer of ownership
Patents	Traffic accidents	Unclaimed property
Promissory notes	Trespass	
Sales contracts	Unfair competition	
Subscriptions		

Inheritance Law	Family Law	Corporation Law
Estates	Adoption	Corporation finance
Probate	Annulment	Documents of incor-
Trusts	Divorce	poration
Wills	Marriage	Mergers and acquisi-
		tions

Excerpted from: World Book Encyclopedia, 1983 edition, volume 12, 120e and 120f.

Federal and state statutes are periodically compiled and published as codes. Federal laws are known as the United States Codes and state laws are referred to as state codes. Most law libraries have a copy of the United States Codes and some or all of the state codes. Statutory law has greatly increased in the past few decades, and—to a large degree—public law is now based on statutory law.

In addition to enacting specific laws, federal, state, and local lawmaking bodies establish executive and administrative agencies to administer programs or accomplish certain goals. These agencies are usually authorized to establish rules and regulations that will enable them to meet their objectives.

Federal agencies, such as the Department of Health and Human Services (HHS), the Federal Trade Commission (FTC), and the Food and Drug Administration (FDA), have established large-scale programs and many rules affecting heath care. Medicare and controlled substances and drug regulations are examples of administrative rules established by these agencies. Similar agencies at the state and local levels are also sources of regulatory law.

Common Law

The other major source of law, and the basis of the original system of law practiced in this country, is legal precedent established by judicial decision. This is referred to as common or judge-made law. Common law decisions are followed by other judges until the precedent is outdated or overruled by a court of higher authority. This principle of common law is called *stare decisis*, which means "the previous decision stands." This principle is followed to ensure the evenhanded administration of justice.

Common law may be altered by judicial decision or by statute. An example of the latter is the statute in every state that those who practice medicine must have a valid license.

In the mid-1800s it was believed that everyone had the inherent right to practice medicine. At the beginning of the 20th century, it was realized that practicing medicine was not a right but a privilege, and a privilege that should be conferred only upon those who could meet certain standards of competence. As a result, licensing statutes were enacted nullifying the common law right of everyone to practice medicine.

Although common law decisions affect both public and private law, their greatest impact today is on private law matters. Likewise, health care delivery is affected by both public law and private law, but it is basically private law—notably contract and tort law—that affects physicians and other health care professionals.

LAWS OF SUBSTANCE AND PROCEDURE

So far, law has been categorized as public or private and statutory or common. It can also be categorized as either substantive or procedural.

Substantive Law

Substantive law describes the rights and responsibilities of parties in legal relationships. Public health laws require health care providers to report certain communicable diseases to state health agencies; private law requires health care providers to have and use reasonable skill in treating patients. Both are examples of substantive law, the primary subject of this book.

Procedural Law

Procedural law is concerned with how substantive law is implemented and how justice is administered. Procedural law sets forth the rules to settle disputes in a fair and just manner. Some people have referred to procedural laws as the "rules of the game;" others have called procedural laws the "rules of warfare!"

Procedural law is based on the adversary process—positioning opposing sides against each other and granting each side the opportunity to prove its story and/or disprove that of the other side. Its goal is to uncover the truth. While not scientific, the adversary process seems to serve the interests of justice better than any other system devised to date. The adversary process may be described as Winston Churchill once described democracy: "the worst form of government except for all those other forms that have been tried from time to time."[2]

COMPETENCY CHECK: TWO

6. State concisely the primary difference between statutory law and common law.

7. How may common laws be changed?

8. State concisely the essential difference between substantive law and procedural law.

COURT SYSTEMS

There are two main court systems in the United States: the federal and the state. Although there are some technical, procedural differences between the two, the main difference is in jurisdiction.

Federal Courts

The federal courts have jurisdiction over disputes when one or more of the following conditions exist:

- The dispute concerns the United States Constitution or a federal law.
- The U.S. government is a party to the dispute.
- The dispute is between or among citizens of different states or between or among different states.
- Another country or one of its citizens is involved in a dispute with a citizen of this country.
- The dispute occurred on or in international waters.

There are three levels of federal courts, along with some courts that have specialized functions (e.g., tax courts).

The lowest level, and usually the first court to try a case, is the district court. There are approximately 100 district courts in this country. The U.S. Court of Appeals occupies the intermediate level in the federal system. The United States is divided into twelve judicial circuits, each of which has one U. S. Court of Appeals. Appellate courts primarily review decisions made in district courts.

The highest federal court is the Supreme Court of the United States, which is the final court of appeals. Usually it agrees to review only appellate court decisions concerning an interpretation of the United States Constitution.

State Courts

The structure of state court systems is similar to the federal system, with trial courts being the lowest level, appellate courts the intermediate level, and a state supreme court as the final court of appeals. The name of the final court of appeals may vary from state to state. State courts have jurisdiction over a wide variety of matters—essentially all matters that do not fall under the jurisdiction of the federal system. Municipal or city courts are usually considered a part of the state system, but often have exclusive jurisdiction over violations of city ordinances. Municipal courts rarely have jurisdiction over civil suits or criminal cases.

COMPETENCY CHECK: THREE

9. True or False: There are three levels of courts in the federal court system: (1) district courts, usually the first court to try a case; (2) appellate courts, which have the authority to review decisions made in district courts; and (3) the U. S. Supreme Court, the court of final appeal.

10. True or False: The court system in most states parallels the federal court system.

SUMMARY

Increasingly, health care professionals are being sued by their patients or their patients' families. This chapter, therefore, has presented an introduction to the law so that providers can become familiar with the sources of law, with the types of law, and with the federal and state court systems. It has also taken a brief look at contemporary medicolegal problems and the reasons why patients sue health care practitioners.

When you have finished this chapter, complete the corresponding chapter in your workbook and then proceed to Chapter Two.

REFERENCES

1. Morris RC The rise of medical liability suits. *JAMA* 1971;215:844.
2. Humes JC. *The Wit and Wisdom of Winston Churchill.* New York, NY. Harper Collins; 1994:28.

2
Licensure and Certification

L icensure and certification are two ways in which, respectively, state governments and health care professional organizations provide safeguards for people who receive care. This chapter includes a discussion of the licensing of health care providers through state practice acts. It also includes a discussion of the certification of health care providers, including allied health professionals, by their professional organizations.

OBJECTIVES

When you have finished this chapter, you will be able to:

1. List at least four basic elements that state medical practice acts have in common.
2. List the three ways in which a health care provider may obtain a license.
3. Cite four reasons why a health care provider may lose a license.
4. Identify at least two differences between licensure and certification.

LICENSURE

In the United States, medical practice acts regulating the practice of medicine existed as far back as colonial times. However, these acts were repealed in the 1800s because of public opinion that the United States Constitution gave *everyone* the right to practice medicine. Consequently, incompetent medical care and quackery became widespread. In response, many states attempted to establish their own regulations. In 1899 the United States Supreme Court decided a case—*Dent v West Virginia*—that upheld a state's right to establish qualifications for individuals who wished to practice medicine. An excerpt from the court's decision follows:

> The power of the State to provide for the general welfare of its people authorizes it to prescribe all such regulations, as in its judgment, will secure or tend to secure them against the consequences of ignorance and incapacity as well as of deception and fraud...The nature and extent of the qualifications required must depend primarily upon the judgment of the State as to their necessity. If they are appropriate to the calling or profession, and attainable by reasonable study or application, no objection to their validity can be raised because of their stringency or difficulty. It is only when they have no relation to such calling or profession, or are unattainable by such reasonable study and application, that they can operate to deprive one of his rights to pursue a lawful vocation.[1]

By the start of the twentieth century, all states had enacted medical practice acts. Periodically, each state updates its act to reflect current medical, legal, and social standards.

Medical Practice Acts

The medical practice acts vary in wording and scope, but share some basic characteristics. Each:

- Defines the practice of medicine.
- Prohibits the practice of medicine without a valid license.
- Establishes prerequisites for licensure.
- Provides for the establishment of a medical examining board and grants the board the authority to examine applicants and issue licenses.
- Stipulates how often and under what condition the license must be renewed.
- Establishes grounds and procedures for suspending, revoking, and refusing to renew licenses.

Prerequisites for Licensure. The practice acts also vary in stipulating prerequisites for licensure, but most require the applicant to:

- have attained the age of majority (the age a person is considered legally capable of being responsible for all his/her activities);
- be of good moral character;
- have the preprofessional education required by that state as well as graduation from an approved medical school;
- have successfully completed an approved internship program or equivalent;
- be a resident of the state;
- have passed the oral and written examinations developed by the board of medical examiners in that state.

Other Methods of Obtaining a License

There are two ways a physician may become licensed other than by fulfilling the prerequisites established by the state legislature and board of medical examiners: reciprocity or endorsement.

Through **reciprocity**, a health care provider already licensed in one state may be granted a license to practice in another state. This license will only be granted, however, if the second state officially recognizes the licensure requirements of the first state as being at least as stringent as its own standards.

In the absence of a formal reciprocity agreement between states, a physician may be granted a license by **endorsement** if the applicant's credentials and license from another state are judged to meet the licensure requirements of the second state.

Unlike licensure by reciprocity, which is automatic if there is a reciprocity agreement between states, licensure by endorsement is granted on a case-by-case basis.

State licenses must be renewed annually or biennially with most states assessing a license renewal fee. Several states now require health care providers to show evidence of participation in continuing education activities as a condition for renewal.

There are generally some exceptions to the requirement of having a valid, current state license in order to practice. These often include treatment provided by:

- An out-of-state physician who gives emergency care.
- A physician establishing residence in a state for the purpose of obtaining a license.
- A physician affiliated with a federal facility (e.g., a Veterans Administration hospital, an armed forces hospital, or the Public Health Service).
- A physician who is employed in research only.

COMPETENCY CHECK: ONE

1. **Name the law enacted by each state that governs the practice of medicine in that state.**

2. **List the ways a physician may be granted a license to practice medicine.**

Revocation and Suspension of Licenses

All medical practice acts set forth grounds and policies for revoking and suspending physicians' licenses. Some acts set forth general grounds, some delineate specific acts, and others give both general and specific actions for which a physician's license may be revoked. In many states, the state board of medical examiners is empowered to revoke licenses; in others, a separate disciplinary body has this authority.

Under no circumstances is a revocation automatic; a physician is always entitled to due process of law, including a written description of charges and a hearing before the appropriate state agency. In most states, decisions rendered by the board or by another authority are subject to appeal through the state's court system.

Several legal scholars have classified the types of misconduct for which physicians might lose their licenses. The following discussion is drawn primarily from categories presented by noted legal scholar Angela Roddy Holder, JD, in *Medical Malpractice Law*. [2]

Classifying offenses makes it easier for the writer to describe them and, it is hoped, for the reader to understand them. Such classifications, however, should not suggest that the practice acts themselves set forth rigid or discrete categories of misconduct. An analysis of the medical practice acts and the decisions rendered under them would show that a criminal offense in one state is considered unprofessional conduct in another, fraud in another, and professional incompetence in another.

Any one of the behaviors described could be grounds for revoking or suspending a license. Allied health professionals must be aware of such offenses in order to fulfill their professional obligations to their employers, patients, and the public, as well as to protect themselves.

The most frequent reason a physician's license is revoked is **conviction of a criminal offense.**

Examples of criminal offenses that have resulted in license revocation include income tax evasion, murder, rape, counterfeiting and violating narcotics laws. As some of these examples suggest, the crime does not have to relate to the practice of medicine to be grounds for revocation.

The number of cases based on violation of narcotics laws has increased substantially in recent years. Gross failure to keep accurate narcotics records is a criminal offense for which an allied health professional may have some liability (See Chapter Nine).

Unprofessional conduct is very broad and somewhat vague, covering a variety of offenses. Some states use the term "gross immorality." Offenses under this heading are considered serious breaches of ethics and morality, which may or may not be criminal offenses.

Unprofessional conduct has been defined as "conduct that would in the common judgment be deemed 'dishonorable' or 'unprofessional.'"[3] It has also been defined as conduct that does not meet the standards of professional behavior accepted by other physicians in the community.[4]

Actual cases culminating in the revocation of a physician's license on the grounds of unprofessional conduct include the willful betrayal of a physician-patient confidence, substance abuse (the most common grounds in this category), sexual misbehavior, and assistance of an unlicensed and untrained person in the practice of medicine.

> A physician employing a bookkeeper permitted him to practice medicine under the physician's direction. The bookkeeper's duties included examining, diagnosing, and treating patients, with fees for these services going to the physician. The physician lost his license to practice on grounds of unprofessional conduct in permitting the bookkeeper to practice medicine. (*Hughes v State Board of Health*, 159 S.W.2d 277, Mo. 1942)

Using discredited drug therapy is usually considered unprofessional conduct, but the legitimate use of new and unproved medication or treatment is not.

Some states consider a **fraudulent act** to be unprofessional conduct, but not as grounds for revoking a license.

In order for an act to be deemed fraudulent, it must be shown that there was an intent to deceive; an honest error or misrepresentation does not constitute a fraudulent act.

A license granted as a result of a fraudulent application is always subject to revocation, provided it can be shown that false answers regarding the physician's qualifications were given on the application. A diploma from a fraudulent medical school, and an application and diploma in someone else's name are examples of fraud.

Other fraudulent acts that could result in revocation of a license include:

- Submitting a bill to a governmental agency claiming that services were rendered when, in fact, they were not. Filing false Medicare or Medicaid forms is also a federal crime.

> A physician submitted claims on four United Medical Service patients, stating he had performed office surgery. Three of the four patients testified that they had never had surgery. The physician claimed the bills were filed as an innocent mistake by his secretary, who had no intent to defraud. The Commissioner of Education suspended the physician's license for six months, a decision upheld by the courts. (*D'Alois v Allen*, 297 N.Y.S.2d 826, 1969)

- Preparing and submitting false medical reports.

  A physician incorrectly diagnosed a patient's disease as syphilis. To avoid admitting this error to the patient, the physician falsely recorded a positive blood test for syphilis on the patient's medical record. The physician's license was revoked for making a fraudulent diagnosis. (*Brown v Hassig*, 15 P.2d 401, Kan. 1932)

- Misrepresenting to the public or to a patient the ability to cure an ailment; advertising a secret cure or special powers.

Some states permit revocation on the basis of **professional incompetence**, negligence, and/or malpractice. Repeated incidents of gross negligence are usually necessary for revocation of a medical license. A single incident of mistaken judgment or ordinary negligence has not resulted in license revocation.

Gross negligence may be defined as conduct suggesting a high disregard for human welfare, conduct of a reckless nature, or failure to use even a minimum degree of care in one's dealings with other people.

Ordinary negligence (a subject discussed thoroughly in Chapter Six) may be defined as the failure to use care that a reasonable person would use.

COMPETENCY CHECK: TWO

3. **True or False: The important difference between an honest mistake and a fraudulent act is that the latter shows there was an intent to deceive.**

4. **True or False: Three categories of offenses for which a physician's license may be revoked in most states are criminal offenses, unprofessional conduct, and fraud.**

Allied Health Professional Licensure

In addition to dentists, physicians, podiatrists, pharmacists, optometrists, and veterinarians, some allied health professionals must have a state license in order to practice in any state.

Many types of health care personnel are required to have a license in some states but not in others.

The proliferation of categories of allied health personnel seeking licensure became a serious problem in the late 1960s and early 1970s. Problems associated with this proliferation included:

1. Poorly defined categories, with designated duties sometimes overlapping licensed and unlicensed occupations.
2. Fragmentation of responsibilities among examining boards, state departments of health, and regulatory authorities.
3. Obstacles to career and geographical mobility for licensees.

The problems became so serious that in 1971 the then Department of Health, Education, and Welfare recommended a two-year moratorium on legislation to create classes of health care personnel subject to state or federal regulation.

The moratorium was subsequently extended for two more years. Its purpose was to provide states, professional organizations, and interested agencies an opportunity to review their licensure and certification policies.

Since the moratorium was recommended, many states and professional organizations have assessed their licensing and certification programs. As a result, there seems to be a trend toward developing and recognizing national standards of competence.

CERTIFICATION OF PHYSICIANS AND ALLIED HEALTH PROFESSIONALS

In addition to having a state license attesting to their competence, many physicians elect to become certified within their chosen specialty. Those who have earned a specialty certificate refer to themselves as "board certified," since the certificate is awarded by a board or body of specialists in the same field.

Each of the recognized medical specialties has organized a national board composed of outstanding physicians in the specialty, and has given the board the responsibilities of developing and administering specialty examinations and issuing certificates to those who pass the examinations. In addition, many allied health professional organizations offer certification programs to practitioners within their fields.

Certification is a voluntary process, and no state requires a physician to be board certified in order to practice. Many hospitals, however, consider certification a prerequisite for physicians seeking staff privileges or for allied health personnel seeking employment.

When a profession is both licensed and certified, the license usually means the licensee has met minimum standards of competence; a certificate indicates that its holder has met a higher standard of competence. Certification standards in unlicensed fields are more difficult to define, because they depend on the goals and objectives of the organization offering the program. The usual goals are to identify competent practitioners and promote the standards of excellence aspired to by the practitioners.

Most organizations offering certification programs are addressing the subject of recertification to encourage or require certificate holders to keep abreast of technological and scientific advancements.

COMPETENCY CHECK: THREE

5. **True or False: Some allied health professionals must have a state license in order to practice.**

6. **True or False: Most states require specialists to be board certified in order to practice.**

Documentation of Education and Training

Educational and training institutions such as colleges, universities, and public or private vocational-technical institutions grant some type of acknowledgment to individuals who complete the required course of study. In these situations, the documentation may be a degree, a diploma, or a certificate. Academic documentation should not be confused with the certification awarded by professional associations.

Fig. 2-A: Comparison of Licensing, Certification, and Academic Documentation

Licensing	Certification	Degree, Diploma, Certificate
Granted by state	Awarded by professional group (usually)	Awarded by educational institution
Mandatory	Voluntary (usually)	Sometimes mandatory, sometimes voluntary
Minimum level competence	Higher level of competence (usually)	Minimum level of competence

SUMMARY

This chapter examined state requirements for licensure and professional association voluntary certification programs.

All physicians must be licensed under state medical practice acts. They may become licensed through examination, reciprocity, or endorsement.

Physicians may have their licenses suspended or revoked as the result of criminal convictions, unprofessional conduct, fraud, or professional incompetence.

Many other health care professionals must be licensed in order to practice. Some health care professionals are required to have licenses in some states, but not in others.

When you have finished reading this chapter, complete the corresponding chapter in your workbook and then proceed to Chapter Three.

REFERENCES

1. Dent v West Virginia, 129 U.S. 114 (1889).
2. Holder AR. *Medical Malpractice Law*, 2nd ed. New York, NY: John Wiley & Sons; 1978:341-351.
3. People v M'Coy, 17 N.E. 786, 787 (Ill. 1888).
4. Board of Medical Examiners of the State of Oregon v Mintz, 378 P.2d 945 (Or. 1963).

3

The Doctor–Patient Relationship

The doctor–patient relationship is the foundation of medical law. Upon it rests the legal rights and obligations of both patients and doctors.

This chapter focuses on the doctor–patient contract and special situations in the doctor–patient relationship.

OBJECTIVES

After studying the legal nature of the doctor–patient relationship in this chapter, you will be able to:

1. List the four elements of a contract.
2. List three rights of patients with regard to obtaining medical treatment.
3. List the rights of doctors with regard to providing medical treatment.
4. Identify the respective obligations of doctors and patients who have established doctor–patient contracts.
5. Explain three ways of terminating the doctor–patient contract.
6. Prepare an effective withdrawal letter.
7. Describe three different types of situations in which a doctor could be charged with abandonment.
8. Define and give examples of the following terms: abandonment, emancipated minor, implied contract, implied limited contract, standard of care, and Good Samaritan law.

THE DOCTOR–PATIENT CONTRACT

The doctor–patient relationship is a contractual one and contains certain elements found in all legal contracts:

1. the offer and acceptance;
2. the consideration;
3. legal capacity to contract; and
4. legal subject matter.

Often during the first visit with the doctor, an individual says literally or by action (the patient's presence usually implies he/she is seeking the doctor's services), "Will you treat me?" This is considered **the offer**.

Next, the doctor either literally or by behavior accepts the patient. Again, just as the patient's offer can be implied by his/her presence, the doctor's **acceptance** can be implied by his/her willingness to provide a service.

Under some circumstances, a doctor might actually make the offer and the patient accept the offer. It really makes no difference which party is the offeror and which party is the offeree. The contract is in effect as long as there is the mutual exchange of promises.

Consideration is the mutual exchange of promises. The doctor promises to treat the patient, and the patient promises to compensate the physician for services rendered. The mutual exchange of promises is often implied by the actions of both parties. The doctor performs a service and the patient accepts it, thereby implying his/her willingness to compensate the doctor for services rendered.

Legal capacity to contract means that the parties are mentally competent adults. Minors and those under legal disability require another person to act on their behalf. The contract must contain **legal subject matter**. A contract would not be valid if it involved breaking a law.

Implied Contracts

Most patients do not refer, during normal conversations, to their "contracts" with doctors. Most doctor–patient contracts are implied, which means the actions and behaviors of both parties indicate that the contract was established. For example: A doctor treats a new, adult patient by injecting a medication. Since the patient did not have to permit the injection and since the doctor was not obligated to give it, the fact that it was provided and accepted implies the establishment of the doctor–patient relationship.

Statute of Frauds

The statute of frauds, a law enacted in every state, stipulates which contracts must be written to be enforceable. In no state does the statute of frauds require the doctor– patient contract to be written; implied doctor–patient contracts are enforceable.

There are two types of contracts relevant to health care that usually must be written to be enforceable: 1) A third-party agreement to be responsible for another's debts; and 2) A contract that will not be completed within one year.

Suppose a patient's friend orally agrees to pay the physician for services rendered to the patient, but does not put this intent in writing. If the friend reneges on this agreement and the patient does not pay, the physician has no legal recourse to recover his/her fees because the agreement was not in writing. The duration of orthodontia commonly exceeds one year. If the agreement between the patient and orthodontist was not written and the patient fails to comply with the terms for payment, the dentist usually has no legal recourse.

COMPETENCY CHECK: ONE

1.   **List the four elements of a contract.**

2.   **Explain "legal capacity to contract."** 2-competent adults

Rights of patients

Under the system of law practiced in the United States, a patient has many rights:

1.   A patient has the right to choose the doctor from whom he/she wishes to receive treatment.

     If a group of doctors has a policy of rotating doctors in the office or on call so that a patient does not always see the doctor of choice, that policy should be clearly stated during the patient's first visit. If the patient doesn't like the policy, he/she may go elsewhere.

2. A patient has the right to determine whether medical treatment will begin and to set limits on the care provided. A mentally competent adult has the right to refuse medical treatment, and, with very few exceptions, neither another person nor the state can force the person to accept treatment. The phrase "right to die" is based on this concept. The concept is exemplified in *Natanson v Kline* (1960):

> It follows that each man is considered to be master of his own body, and he may, if he be of sound mind, expressly prohibit the performance of life-saving surgery, or other medical treatment. A doctor might well believe that an operation or form of treatment is desirable or necessary but the law does not permit him to substitute his own judgment for that of the patient by any form of artifice or deception.[1]

3. A patient has the right to know before treatment begins what it shall consist of, what effect it will have on his/her body, and what dangers are inherent in it. These concepts are sometimes summed up by the expression "the patient has a right to give an informed consent to treatment." This subject is more thoroughly discussed in Chapter Five.

Patients' Obligations

Once the doctor–patient relationship is established, each party incurs certain obligations. The patient has three obligations in this contract.

1. The patient is obliged to tell the doctor the truth about the nature and duration of symptoms and to provide an accurate and thorough medical history. Failure to do so could adversely affect the doctor's

ability to diagnose and treat the patient's illness. It could also jeopardize the patient's cause for legal action against the doctor in a subsequent lawsuit alleging negligent treatment.

A father took his young child to a hospital emergency room after the child had swallowed an unknown quantity of aspirin. The emergency room attendants told the father to be sure to tell the doctor (who would examine the child) about the aspirin. The father did not do so. The doctor's diagnosis was the flu, and the child died. The parents sued for negligent misdiagnosis. The court found for the defendant doctor, noting that he could not be held responsible for the father's failure to inform. *(Johnson v St. Paul Mercury Insurance Company,* 219 So.2d 524, La. 1969)

2. The patient is expected to follow the doctor's instructions concerning diet, medication, exercise, habits, follow-up appointments, etc. The patient who leaves the hospital without the doctor's permission, or in opposition to the doctor's instructions, is not meeting his/her responsibilities in the doctor–patient relationship.

   The patient is relieved of his/her obligation only if he/she believes, for good reason, that the doctor's instructions are not in accord with sound medical practice.

   Suppose, for example, a doctor inadvertently prescribed a drug to which the patient was allergic. The patient knew he/she was allergic to the drug, but took it anyway. He/she suffered a reaction and then sued the doctor for negligence. This is a hypothetical case and we can only surmise what the courts would decide. The court would probably find for the doctor, however, because the patient knew that he/she would suffer the drug reaction.

3. A patient is obligated to pay the doctor for services rendered. Nonpayment, however, does not affect the establishment or existence of the contract and does not relieve either party of other responsibilities. The patient who fails to pay for services may be sued

for breach of contract, although this practice is discouraged because it tends to provoke lawsuits against doctors.

Rights of Doctors

Doctors in private practice also have certain rights. They have the right to accept patients of their own choosing and to refuse service to new patients or to former patients with new problems.

There is one exception to the right of doctors to refuse service. When a doctor agrees to accept anyone who seeks treatment with a particular condition or in a particular locale, that doctor is legally obligated to accept all people who meet the stipulated criteria. For example, doctors with hospital staff privileges are often required by the hospitals to periodically provide emergency room service. While on emergency room duty, a doctor cannot refuse service to any emergency patients brought to that hospital.

Similarly, doctors hired expressly to provide emergency room service, as well as interns and residents assigned there, are obliged to provide emergency service to all patients requiring it.

> A patient was brought to a hospital emergency room with a severe gunshot wound in his chest. The physician on call came and looked at the patient, but did not provide first aid, even though he realized the patient was in shock. Instead, the doctor ordered the man transferred to another hospital. The patient died in the ambulance en route. The court ruled that the doctor was liable for not treating the patient. (*New Biloxi Hospital, Inc. v Frazier*, 146 So.2d 882, Miss. 1962)

Doctors also have the right to stipulate the types of services they will give and how they will be provided.

> The patient of an obstetrician asked that her baby be delivered at home. The obstetrician refused. The woman terminated the relationship, indicating that she would hire a midwife. Complications developed during the woman's labor, and the obstetrician was asked to come to the home. He refused, but said he would deliver the baby if the woman was brought to the

hospital. Six hours later the woman arrived, but the baby was delivered dead. When the parents sued the obstetrician, the court dismissed the case, noting that the dangers of a home delivery are obvious and that the obstetrician had the right to refuse service under the circumstances. (*Vidrine v Mayes*, 127 So.2d 809, La. 1961)

Doctors may specialize, may open offices where they choose, and may set office hours.

A patient cut her leg and contacted a doctor for treatment. After she was treated, the doctor told her to return for follow-up care in two days. Instead, the patient left on vacation. Complications developed and she called the doctor to insist that he come and treat her at the vacation site. He refused and the patient sued him. The court ruled the physician was entitled to limit his practice to the community. (*McNamara v Emmons*, 97 P.2d 503, Cal. 1939)

Doctors have the right to change their services and change how those services are provided. They also have the right to take vacations, and to change locations and times of availability. They must, however, give patients reasonable notice of any such changes. Obstetricians must be especially careful to notify patients of any changes in availability. Doctors must make arrangements for qualified substitutes to care for their patients during times of unavailability.

Doctors' Obligations

As indicated above, once the doctor–patient relationship is established, each party incurs certain obligations. Many of the doctor's obligations are summed up by the statement, "the patient is owed the standard of care."

"Standard of care" means the care provided by a doctor who has and uses reasonable skill, experience, and knowledge in treating the patient. "Reasonable," as usually defined by the courts, means that the doctor's skills, experience, and knowledge must be average when compared to like doctors in the same circumstances.

"Like" doctors are doctors in the same specialty. "Same circumstances" usually means access to same or similar equipment and facilities; in some cases, the term means the same or similar community.

Once the doctor–patient relationship is established, the doctor is obliged to:

- Treat the patient as long as the condition requires, or until a proper withdrawal or discharge is made.
- Inform patients of proposed treatment and obtain appropriate consent before proceeding.
- Caution patients against unneeded or undesirable surgery.
- Give complete and accurate instructions to the patient and, when applicable, to the person responsible for the patient in the doctor's absence.
- Respect the patient's privacy and confidential information acquired during the course of the doctor–patient relationship.

A doctor is *not* obligated to:

- Accept new patients or former patients with new problems.
- Demonstrate perfect judgment, acquire a maximum level of skill, obtain the greatest amount of education.
- Correctly diagnose every medical problem or cure each patient.
- Return a patient to the state of health experienced before the patient became ill or injured.
- Know in advance how each patient will respond to every drug or anesthetic.
- Continue treating a patient who has discharged the doctor, even if the patient later has adverse effects.

Guarantees

Usually, the doctor guarantees only that he/she has reasonable skill, experience, and knowledge, and will exercise them diligently.

Although prudence would caution against it, a doctor is not forbidden to make guarantees. He/she may promise the patient complete recovery, no permanent side effects, and total satisfaction with the results. A doctor may also promise that only certain drugs or procedures will be used in treatment. Such promises are legally binding, and if they are not kept, the doctor may be liable for breach of contract, even if the standard of care was met or exceeded. In a breach of contract suit, the plaintiff simply has to show that the defendant did not meet the terms of their agreement.

> A patient required surgery for an ulcer. The surgeon described the operation as simple and as a cure-all, and he told the patient he would be able to return to work in two to four weeks. Complications developed during surgery, and the patient had to have three more operations. He also developed serum hepatitis from a blood transfusion. The patient sued the surgeon for breach of contract to cure, and the court found for the patient. (*Guilmet v Campbell*, 188 N.W.2d 601, Mich.1971)

Overly optimistic statements about a patient's prognosis could be misinterpreted as a promise to cure. Regarding therapeutic procedures, most courts realize that some comments are meant to reassure an anxious patient, and they permit doctors latitude in the remarks they make to patients. Regarding elective procedures, especially cosmetic surgery, courts are apt to hold a doctor to any promises made.

COMPETENCY CHECK: TWO

3. Explain the following statement: A doctor is obligated to provide each patient with the standard of care.

4. List three specific obligations a doctor owes a patient.

5. Explain what the doctor guarantees the patient when establishing an implied contract.

6. List three of the patient's contractual obligations.

TERMINATION OF CONTRACT

Once the doctor–patient relationship is established, the doctor is obliged to treat the patient until: 1) his/her condition

no longer requires treatment; 2) the doctor expressly withdraws from the case; or 3) the patient discharges the doctor.

Usually the contract is terminated when the patient no
longer requires the doctor's services.

Under these circumstances, the contract is terminated
by implication; the patient no longer needs medical treatment and does not seek it.

Sometimes, the contract is terminated *during* treatment.
If the patient does not follow instructions, breaks appointments, or leaves the hospital against the doctor's advice, the
doctor may want to withdraw from the case.

Conversely, the patient may be dissatisfied with the
treatment or with some other aspect of care and either tells
the doctor his/her services are no longer wanted or simply
stops seeking treatment from that doctor.

Abandonment

A doctor who withdraws from a case without properly terminating the relationship may be sued for abandonment.
Abandonment has been defined as " . . . the unilateral severance by the doctor of the professional relationship between himself and the patient without reasonable notice, at
a time when there is still the necessity of continuing medical attention."[2]

A charge of abandonment may arise from several different types of situations:

1. The doctor abruptly and without reasonable notice
   stops treating a patient whose condition requires
   additional or continued care.

   A doctor decided it was necessary to use forceps in the
   delivery of a baby. The woman, who had been in labor a
   long time, became hysterical when she saw the instrument,
   and the doctor had to stop. After this happened two more
   times, the doctor told her "You quit your screaming. If you
   don't quit, I'll quit." Then he abruptly left the patient's
   house and refused to return. The patient sued the doctor
   for abandonment. The court ruled in her favor and said,
   "Such conduct evidenced a wanton disregard not only of

professional ethics, but of the terms of his actual contract." (*Lathrope v Flood*, 63 P.1007, Cal. 1901)

After having varicose vein surgery by one surgeon, the patient's leg became gangrenous. The surgeon's partner recommended immediate amputation of the patient's foot and offered to do it. The patient consented and expected the operation to be performed immediately. Four days passed without the patient seeing or hearing from the partner, so he had himself transferred to another hospital for the surgery. The patient sued the surgeon's partner for abandonment, and the court held that the question of abandonment by the physician was a question of fact that should be submitted to the jury. (*McGulpin v Bessmer*, 43 N.W.2d 121, Iowa 1950)

2. The doctor fails to see the patient as often as the patient's condition requires or he/she incorrectly advises the patient that there is no need for more treatment. (Generally, suits resulting from this situation are tried as professional negligence cases.)

A man with a chronic heart condition was under the care of a doctor. When he became ill one day, the patient's wife called the doctor who had him admitted to the hospital. The doctor, however, did not see the patient for several days and did not order any treatment. The man, who was critically ill, was finally seen by the doctor, but it was too late. The patient died soon after the doctor's visit. His widow sued the doctor, and the court ruled that abandonment had occurred. (*Levy v Kirk*, 187 So.2d 401, Fla. 1966)

3. The doctor fails to provide a qualified substitute doctor during his/her absence. Doctors are obligated to arrange for a qualified substitute to care for their patients in their absence. The substitute's qualifications must be equal to or better than those of the doctor for whom he/she is substituting.

A doctor had his patient admitted to a hospital and scheduled her for an arteriogram. Before it could be performed, the doctor became ill and left town to recuperate. His associate saw the patient, explained the situation, and offered her the option of permitting him to do the procedure or postponing it until her physician's return. She asked the associate to perform it. She suffered a stroke and then sued the first physician for abandonment. The court ruled that since the associate was qualified, abandonment had not occurred. (*Kenney v Piedmont Hospital*, 222 S.E.2d 162, Ga. 1975)

Obstetricians are especially prone to charges of abandonment, since a baby's arrival can seldom be scheduled or accurately predicted. Also, the treatment of one patient does not justify a doctor's failure to fulfill obligations to another.

In preparation for a home delivery, a doctor gave his patient some medicine to induce labor. He told the patient that, since it would be at least four hours before she delivered, he would return to his office. Three hours later the woman's pains became severe. Her husband tried in vain to reach the physician, who had been called to treat another woman in labor. Another physician delivered the baby, who died a few minutes later. The patient sued the first physician for abandonment. In reversing a directed verdict for the defendant and awarding the plaintiff a new trial, the court said the physician had a duty to remain with the patient or to provide a qualified substitute. (*Young v Jordan*, 145 S.E.41, W.Va. 1928)

Withdrawal by physician

If the physician wishes to withdraw from the care of a patient, the following procedure should be followed:

1. Prepare a letter containing the following elements:

   - A statement that the provider is withdrawing and a sufficient explanation for the withdrawal.
   - A recommendation, if appropriate, that the patient seek continued medical treatment.
   - An offer to provide the patient's new caregiver with information in his/her medical records.
   - The provider's signature.

2. Send the letter certified mail, to addressee only, with return receipt requested.

3. Place a copy of the letter and the returned receipt in the patient's file to show when it was sent.

Figure 3-A. Sample Letters of Withdrawal

Form 1a

Date: _____

Dear _____:

I will no longer be able to provide medical care to (you/your children). If you require medical care within the next __ days I will be available, but in no event longer than __ days.

To assist you in continuing to receive medical care for (you/your children), we will make records available to a new physician as soon as you authorize us to send them to that physician.

Sincerely,

_____, M.D.

Form 1b

Date:_____

Dear: _____:

I find it necessary to inform you that I am withdrawing from further professional attendance upon you because you have persisted in refusing to follow my medical advice and treatment. Since your condition requires medical attention, I suggest that you place yourself under the care of another physician without delay. If you desire, I shall be available to attend you for a reasonable time after you receive this letter, but in no event for more than___ days.

This should give you ample time to select a physician of your choice from the many competent practitioners in this city. With your authorization, I will make available to this physician your case history and information regarding the diagnosis and treatment you have received from me.

Very truly yours,

_____, M.D.

Discharge by patient

If the health care provider is discharged by the patient, the patient should send a letter to the provider indicating the dismissal. If a patient verbally discharges a provider, but does not follow up in writing, the physician should send a letter to the patient confirming the dismissal.

This procedure is recommended for protecting the provider in case it becomes necessary to show that the provider did not abandon the patient but was discharged. In the confirming letter, the provider should reiterate the discharge and follow the previously outlined procedure.

COMPETENCY CHECK: THREE

7. When a doctor decides to withdraw from a case because the patient is not following instructions, what specific action should the doctor take?

8. If a patient discharges a doctor, why should the doctor confirm the discharge in writing?

SPECIAL SITUATIONS

The previous sections discussed the general obligations of both parties to the doctor–patient relationship. The following paragraphs look at special situations in the relationship.

Treatment of Minors

Occasionally doctors utilize their medical expertise at the request of someone other than the patient. This most commonly occurs when a parent requests treatment for a minor child. Although the child is the patient and the recipient of care, the parent is legally responsible for meeting the patient's obligations to the doctor.

An exception is the emancipated minor—a minor child who has voluntarily left his/her parents' home for the purpose of supporting himself/herself and living independently.[3] An emancipated minor is responsible for his/her own debts.

A teenage girl was employed, self-supporting and living with friends away from her parents' home. She was admitted to a hospital for surgery. The hospital required the girl's father to sign the consent form, which he did. He refused, however, to sign a form accepting financial responsibility for the girl's hospital bill. When the bill was not paid, the hospital sued the father. The court found him not liable because the girl was an "emancipated minor." (*Ison v Florida Sanitarium and Benevolent Ass'n*, 302 So.2d 200, Fla. 1974)

Good Samaritan Laws

[handwritten annotation: - designed to protect med. personnel from law suits when tx is rendered at Scene - provided rendered in good faith]

Within the past twenty years, most states have enacted Good Samaritan laws to encourage health care providers to provide medical assistance at the scene of accidents or emergencies without fear of being sued for negligence. These statutes vary greatly but have in common the intent to eliminate recovery of damages for ordinary negligence in the course of medical treatment at the scene of an accident. Gross negligence, on the other hand, is usually not exempted.

Implied Limited Contracts

When a doctor renders emergency treatment in a situation not covered by a special arrangement, such as in an emergency room, the doctor–patient relationship is usually limited to treatment provided at the site of the emergency and is based on the victim's implied request for treatment. The law's position is that the victim in an emergency where immediate treatment is required to save the person's life or to prevent serious medical consequences would naturally request treatment from the doctor if he/she were able. Therefore, the request for treatment can be implied, as must be the promise to compensate the doctor for services rendered.

The doctor providing emergency care is not obligated to treat the patient until the medical problem is completely resolved. Rather, the doctor's obligation is limited to providing emergency treatment until the victim is turned over to competent medical authority.

During the time the limited implied contract is in effect, the doctor's obligations are the same as those in any doctor–patient contract; that is, the doctor is obligated to have and use reasonable skill, knowledge, and experience. Of course, a doctor without proper equipment and drugs could not provide the same quality of care at the scene of an accident that he/she or any other doctor could provide in an office or hospital. Should a lawsuit alleging negligence arise, the patient would have to show that the doctor's care was below the standard of care that would have been provided by like doctors in similar circumstances.

COMPETENCY CHECK: FOUR

9. What can a physician who withdraws from a case without giving the patient proper notice be sued for?

10. What can a physician who does not arrange for a qualified substitute to care for his/her patients during times of his/her unavailability be sued for?

11. Who is responsible for the medical bills of an emanicipated minor?

12. In what way is the physician–patient relationship established at the scene of an accident limited?

Assessment Examinations

Another fairly common situation in which the doctor utilizes expertise at the request of someone other than the patient occurs when a doctor examines a person solely to assess the patient's physical condition, with no intent of advising or providing treatment.

Examples include doctors hired by insurance companies to examine potential policyholders or claimants, doctors employed by companies to perform preemployment physicals, and doctors appointed by the courts to examine litigants.

In most states, the doctor–patient relationship is not established in such instances because the party being examined is not requesting medical advice or treatment and the doctor is not offering it.

> X-rays taken of a job applicant during a preemployment physical indicated that the applicant had tuberculosis. The applicant was hired but not told of the x-ray findings. Several years later she became seriously ill with tuberculosis and sued the doctor and employer. The court ruled that no doctor–patient relationship had been established at the time of the preemployment physical and, therefore, the doctor was not obligated to report the x-ray findings to the patient. (*Lotspeich v Chance Vought Aircraft*, 369 S.W.2d 705, Tex. 1963)

In most states a doctor performing an assessment examination is under no obligation to inform the examinee of the findings or results. All the reports go to the individual or company ordering and paying for the examination.

Recently, however, there have been decisions that indicate the law may be changing. A few states now require doctors performing assessment examinations to report the results to the examinee. The doctor is not obligated to provide treatment, but is obligated to provide the information.

The following scenario is illustrative of how this principle of law is changing:

> In 1985, Sidney Green saw Dr. Leslie T. Walker at the direction of his employer. He was examined and tests run; he was pronounced fit without restriction. About a year later, cancer was diagnosed and he died soon after filing a lawsuit against Dr. Walker for his failure to diagnose the case. Walker's attorney argued that even if there had been a spot on the x-ray, the exam was done for Green's employer and, therefore, there was no doctor–patient relationship. The verdict was in the doctor's favor.
>
> Mrs. Green appealed. In 1990 the federal court of appeals ruled in her favor; the jury found the doctor liable. The appellate court was guided by a 1988 case in Louisiana. The court ruled that although there may not be the creation of the usual doctor–patient relationship, that does not mean that the physician has no duty toward the person being examined. Physicians must approach company examinations with the same degree of care they'd exercise with a private patient.[4]

SUMMARY

The physician–patient relationship is of fundamental importance in medical law and ethics. It is the foundation upon which rests the legal rights and obligations of both physician and patient.

In this chapter you learned about the basic rights of patients and physicians in the health care delivery system. You also learned about the rights and obligations inherent in the physician–patient contract.

The patient's basic rights include the right to:

- choose the provider from whom he/she wishes to receive treatment;
- say whether treatment will be accepted and what limits will be put on that treatment; and
- know before treatment begins what it shall consist of, its effects, and any inherent dangers.

The physician's basic rights include the right to:

- Accept patients of his/her own choosing.
- Stipulate the type of service he/she will provide and how it will be provided.
- Specialize.
- Open offices at a place and time of his/her own choosing.

Under the contract, both the physician and the patient have certain obligations.

The patient is obligated to:

- Tell the physician about the nature and duration of the symptoms and about his/her medical history.
- Follow the physician's instructions.
- Pay the physician for services rendered.

The physician must provide "the standard of care." Included in this are the following explicit obligations:

- Treat the patient as long as his/her condition requires it, or until withdrawal or discharge.
- Inform the patient of proposed treatment and obtain informed consent before proceeding.
- Caution the patient against unneeded or undesirable surgery.
- Give complete and accurate information to the patient.
- Respect the patient's privacy.

The physician is *not* obligated to:

- Accept new patients or former patients with new problems.
- Demonstrate perfect skill or infallible judgment.
- Diagnose every medical problem accurately.
- Return a patient to his/her original state of health.
- Know in advance how each patient will respond to treatment.
- Continue treating a patient after he/she has been discharged.

The contract may be terminated in one of three ways—as a result of no need for further treatment, withdrawal by the physician, or discharge by the patient. Should the physician withdraw, he/she should properly terminate the relationship in writing, giving a reasonable termination date. Should the physician be discharged, he/she should confirm the termination of the contract in writing.

There are some instances in which someone other than the patient requests the physician's services—parents requesting treatment for a minor child, for example, or an insurance company requesting an assessment examination.

There are also situations in which a physician–patient relationship has not actually been established or has been established only on a limited basis. The assessment examination is an example of the former. Emergency treatment is an example of the latter. During the time the limited relationship or contract is in effect, the physician's obligations are the same as they are in any physician–patient contract. However, because of the circumstances surrounding emergency care, many states have enacted Good Samaritan laws to encourage physicians to provide medical assistance without fear of being sued for negligence or abandonment.

When you have finished reading this chapter, complete the corresponding chapter in your workbook and then proceed to Chapter Four.

REFERENCES

1. Natanson v Kline, 350 P.2d 1093 (Kan. 1960).
2. Morris RC., Mortiz AR. *Doctor and Patient and the Law*. 5th ed. St. Louis, Mo: CV Mosby Company; 1971:49.
3. Holder AR. *Medical Malpractice Law*, 2nd ed. New York, NY: John Wiley and Sons; 1978:8.
4. Murray D. Don't get burned doing company physicals. *Medical Economics*. August 19, 1991;68:90-91.

4

Confidentiality in the Doctor–Patient Relationship

The doctor–patient relationship is confidential. Information that doctors and their employees acquire about patients must not be disclosed to any third party unless the patient consents or unless disclosure is required by law.

OBJECTIVES

After studying this chapter on the confidential nature of this relationship, on legally required disclosures, and on the patient's right to privacy, you will be able to:

1. Identify the legal basis of the principle of confidentiality.
2. Prepare a legally-binding form authorizing the disclosure of confidential patient information to a third party.
3. State the purpose of privileged communication statutes.
4. List four precautions health professionals should take to reduce the possibility of inadvertently infringing on the patient's right to confidentiality.
5. Define the following terms: *subpoena, subpoena duces tecum*, and privileged communication.

DOCTOR–PATIENT COMMUNICATIONS

As discussed in Chapter Three, patients are obliged to tell doctors the truth about their symptoms and their medical history. To help patients feel comfortable in telling the truth and to reduce their fears that the information will become public, all doctors take an oath that they will keep patient information confidential.

The confidentiality of patient information is a long-recognized principle of the medical profession. According to historical records, it was first expressed by Hippocrates in the fifth century B.C. The oath physicians take is known as the *Hippocratic Oath.*

Legal Basis of Confidentiality

Because of the emphasis on confidentiality in the Hippocratic Oath, many people believe the confidentiality of the doctor–patient relationship is solely an ethical matter. While betraying a professional confidence is certainly unethical, it is also unlawful.

The confidentiality of doctor–patient communications is recognized as a principle of common law. Most courts permit a patient to sue a doctor for breach of confidence if the unauthorized disclosure was damaging to the patient (See Chapter Eight).

Many states have enacted a statute stipulating that betrayal of a professional secret is grounds for suspending or revoking a doctor's license to practice medicine. In the state of Michigan, for example, an unauthorized disclosure is considered a misdemeanor, punishable by fine, imprisonment, or both.

Authorization to Disclose Information

Medical information about patients is disclosed on a daily basis. With the exception of circumstances described later, physicians should always obtain their patients' written authorizations before sharing any information with any third party.

The Office of the General Counsel, American Medical Association, has prepared several example forms concerning the release of medical information. One is shown in Figure 4-A. Other examples are available from the American Medical Association.

Figure 4-A. Sample Authorization for Disclosure of Information by Patient's Physician

1. I authorize Dr. _____ to disclose complete information to _____ concerning his/her medical findings and treatment of the undersigned from on or about _____ 19 ___ until date of the conclusion of such treatment.

2. Further, I authorize him/her to testify, without limitation, as to all of his/her medical findings and the treatment administered to the undersigned, in any legal action, suit, or proceedings to which I am, or may become a party and I waive on behalf of myself and any persons who may have an interest in the matter, all provisions of law relating to the disclosure of confidential medical information

Witness _____

Signed _____
Place _____
Date _____

Source: Medicolegal Forms with Legal Analysis, *1973 ed, published by the American Medical Association. Reprinted with Permission.*

Each form requires the insertion of information specifying what data can be released and to whom. Note the information required in the first paragraph of the form shown: the name of the doctor being authorized to release the information, the name of the intended recipient, and date on which treatment began.

The inclusion of a date serves to limit the information being released to the treatment of a certain condition. Patients may limit disclosure to a certain condition, but they may not select only certain pieces of information about that condition for release. In other words, patients may authorize either full disclosure or no disclosure, but not partial disclosure.

The second paragraph in the authorization form shown contains two basic statements concerning the patient's legal right to confidentiality. One authorizes the doctor to testify, and the other waives the patient's right to confidentiality with respect to the intended recipient of the information.

The patient's signature, date and place of signing, and the signature of a witness are elements that would help to verify the authenticity of the patient's authorization, if that became necessary.

The patient's authorization to disclose information to one party never implies authorization to disclose such information to another. Each time the patient requests the disclosure of information, a separate authorization form should be completed, signed by the patient, and filed in the medical record.

The right to have information disclosed or kept secret belongs to the patient. The doctor may not refuse to disclose information if disclosure is properly authorized.

Faxing Patient Information

Facsimile (fax) machines have brought advantages to the American economy, including the health care sector.

> The facsimile (fax) machine has secured an important position in health care communications. Within the health care facility, patient care is enhanced when clinical information, such as consultation reports or diagnostic test results, is readily available to a health care practitioner. Such data can be transmitted immediately by fax to the patient care center or doctor's office. The fax may be used between health care facilities to make clinical information immediately available for patient care across the country when a patient becomes ill away from home.
>
> However, the fax machine also opens up avenues for loss of patient confidentiality and impacts medical record integrity.[1]

Fax transmissions should be used between health care facilities only when the information is needed immediately for a patient visit. Routine transfer of patient information to attorneys, insurance companies, or other health care facilities should be handled by regular mail or messenger services. Within a facility, the actual patient record should be used.

Each facility needs to develop a written policy concerning the use of fax machines. The following are a couple of the questions to be considered: 1) Under what circumstances should the fax be used? 2) Should a fax used for internal transmission of patient information be destroyed, added to the patient record, or returned to the medical record department?

The American Health Information Management Association (AHIMA) has proposed guidelines for the following concerns:

- How can patient confidentiality be maintained for incoming fax transmissions? The fax machine needs to be located in an area of restricted access with a staff member authorized to receive and distribute faxes related to patient care.
- Can a fax transmission be a legal part of the patient record? How can patient record integrity and quality of documentation be preserved? Incomplete information, omissions, and illegible entries can cause questions about the validity and value of records used in court. Legally, a fax may be part of the patient record, but if the fax is received on thermal paper, a photocopy must be made for the record since the thermal copy will fade.
- How can the authenticity of signatures be verified? Patient signatures should be verified with another sample of the patient's signature; if doctors are going to fax orders, a register with the doctors' signatures may be used to authenticate fax signatures.

COMPETENCY CHECK: ONE

1. List five elements contained in a legally effective form authorizing a doctor to release patient medical information.

2. A patient has been treated by her podiatrist for a number of problems during the past ten years. Most recently she was treated for injuries suffered in an automobile accident. She authorized her podiatrist to disclose the extent of her injuries and treatment received to the other driver's insurance company. How may she limit disclosure to accident-related treatment of her foot?

Privileged Communication Statutes

States have further protected the confidentiality of the doctor–patient relationship by enacting privileged communication statutes (known in some states as a testimonial statute).

The statutes prohibit a doctor from testifying in court about a patient unless the patient specifically consents to the testimony or waives the right to secrecy. Depending on state law, a patient may waive the right to secrecy by testifying voluntarily or by suing the doctor.

The wording and scope of privileged communication statutes vary markedly. In some states, the statutes prohibit doctors from testifying only in civil actions. In other states, the statutes prohibit doctors from testifying in any court proceeding, criminal or civil, except when the patient is involved in a homicide or offers a defense of insanity.

The presence of a third party during communications between doctor and patient may or may not nullify the privileged status of the communication. If the third person is necessary for assisting the doctor, or in aiding communication between doctor and patient, or if the third party is the spouse or a close relative of the patient, the communication remains privileged. Despite many differences, courts do agree on one point: Privileged communication statutes are meant to protect the patient. The patient is entitled to say whether his/her doctor may testify. The doctor may neither refuse to testify if the patient consents, nor testify if the patient does not so authorize.

LEGALLY REQUIRED DISCLOSURES

The patient's right to confidentiality is not absolute. Situations arise in which the public's right to certain information supersedes an individual's right to secrecy. These disclosures can be categorized as disclosures which are:

- Required by subpoena.
- Required by statute to protect public health or welfare.

- Necessary to protect the welfare of the patient or a third party.

Disclosures Required by Subpoena

In those states that do not have a privileged communication statute or in situations in which the information is not considered privileged, a doctor must release patient information when ordered by a court. The order is usually in the form of a *subpoena*, a court order directed to a certain person that requires attendance for testifying at a certain time and place. A subpoena may or may not require a doctor to bring a patient's medical records. However, when the record is required, a *subpoena duces tecum* is usually served. (The literal translation of *subpoena duces tecum* is "under penalty you shall take it with you.")

Occasionally, the allied health professional responsible for the doctor's office records is served with a *subpoena duces tecum*. This subpoena may require the employee either to appear in court at a certain time and with the pertinent records, or—if attorneys on both sides agree—make photocopies of the medical records. In the latter case, the employee should also submit a statement, properly notarized, that the medical records are complete and accurate, and were made by the doctor during the course of treating the patient.

Disclosures Required by Statute to Protect Health or Welfare

All states require health care providers to report certain patient information to appropriate health or law enforcement authorities. When a report is statutorily required, the provider's duty to comply with the law preempts the patient's right to confidentiality.

The full scope of the provider's public duties and responsibilities is explained in Chapter Nine, but those affecting the confidentiality of the provider–patient relationship are mentioned briefly here.

By statute or by regulation, every state and the District of Columbia require health care providers to report to a specified person or agency the following public health and welfare matters:

- vital statistics such as births and deaths;
- injuries due to acts such as gunshots, stabbings, or domestic violence;
- contagious, infectious, or communicable diseases as specified in the applicable statutes and/or regulations. All states require the reporting of sexually transmitted diseases, tuberculosis, hepatitis, and polio, to name a few; and
- known drug addicts. (Federal and state narcotics laws are discussed in Chapter Nine.)

Disclosures to Protect the Welfare of the Patient or Third Party

Health professionals are sometimes confronted with circumstances requiring them to consider, on one hand, the patient's right to secrecy and, on the other hand, another individual's right to know. It is in this area that decisions to release information are most often challenged. It is also this area that generates the greatest number of suits alleging either inappropriate disclosure or negligence in not disclosing. Before the discovery of modern drugs that prevent or control most contagious and communicable diseases, doctors had a positive duty to warn their patients and others in close proximity about the dangerous nature of the diseases. Failure to do so resulted in injury to others, as well as in lawsuits against doctors by people who should have been warned about the contagious nature of a patient's disease.

The following case illustrates the principle that, in some circumstances, the provider's duty to protect public welfare exceeds a patient's right to confidentiality.

A patient was given a preliminary diagnosis of syphilis and advised by his doctor to immediately move out of the small hotel in which he resided until the diagnosis could be verified.

When the doctor learned the next day that the patient had not moved, he told the proprietor that the patient had a "contagious disease." The proprietor made the patient leave. The preliminary diagnosis was later proved incorrect, and the patient sued the doctor for breach of confidence. The court ruled that, under the circumstances, the doctor had the duty to disclose the information. *(Simonsen v Swenson*, 177 N.W.831, Neb. 1920)

In several other cases, this principle has been applied to situations involving psychiatrists and psychologists treating patients with violent inclinations caused by mental problems. In some cases, patients have told their therapists of plans to harm a third party. When the therapist failed to confine the patient or warn the third party, and the patient subsequently carried out the threat, the courts have held the therapist responsible. This reaffirms the principle that a health care professional has a legal and moral responsibility to protect public welfare as well as the welfare of patients.

The following case garnered a lot of media attention:

A student being treated by a university health center psychologist told the psychologist he intended to murder his former girlfriend. The psychologist believed him and made arrangements to have the student hospitalized. The Chief of Service at the hospital ordered the student released, and the student carried out his threat against the girl. Her parents sued the university for either not hospitalizing the student or not warning the girl or her parents of the threat. The court upheld the parents' cause of action. (*Tarasoff v Board of Regents of University of California*, 529 P.2d 553; Cal. 1974)

The courts have also upheld on several occasions a doctor's right to disclose information to another person or agency attempting to help the patient. For example, as long as no malice is involved, a child's doctor could disclose pertinent medical information about the child to a school psychologist without fear of being charged with breach of confidence.

Even when health care practitioners believe that their duty to disclose information outweighs their duty to keep it secret, they must use discretion. In general, confidential information should be:

1. Given in good faith, with reasonable care taken to ensure its accuracy.
2. Reported fairly.
3. Limited to what is necessary for the sake of protection.
4. Given only to the people who need it for the purpose of protection.

Members of the Health Care Team

All health care personnel are legally and ethically bound to respect the privacy of the patient. The ability to keep patient information confidential is a prerequisite for being a member of the health care team.

Handling requests for confidential information is a part of the daily routine for members of the health care team. Well-meaning friends or relatives call to ask how their friend or relative is doing. Attorneys, insurance companies, and employers write or call to request medical information on patient histories, health status, or treatment. All such inquiries must be handled carefully and, of course, according to the doctor's instructions.

Some doctors prefer to handle telephone inquiries about patients themselves and instruct their employees to take the caller's name and number and inform the caller that the doctor will return the call when available. Many other doctors authorize their personnel to handle the calls in accordance with the legal principles outlined in this book and with the doctor's personal instructions and style.

Individuals delegated this enormous and important responsibility must have a clear understanding of their legal obligations and the expectations of their employer.

The facility policy concerning confidentiality should be reviewed with employees annually, and employees should sign a confidentiality statement each year.

Guidelines for Inexperienced Team Members

The following discussion and guidelines are included to help the inexperienced professional apply some of the legal principles discussed in this chapter to everyday situations. It is also an excellent review for all health care personnel.

- Telephone inquiries pose special problems, especially when the voice of the caller is not recognized. Under normal circumstances, the employee taking the call should insist that the caller put the request in writing and include with it the patient's written authorization to disclose the information. If the caller refuses, the assistant should obtain the caller's name, telephone number, and relationship to the patient. The employee should then inform the caller that the doctor will return the call when he/she is available.
- Inquiries from well-meaning friends and relatives of the patient should be politely but firmly refused. In some instances, the doctor may want to discuss the case with a patient's relative, but that is a decision to be made by the doctor.
- Most legitimate inquiries from insurance companies, attorneys, employers, etc., are made in writing and accompanied by the patient's written authorization to disclose the requested information. The authorization form (or copy of it) should be filed in the patient's medical record. Normally it is the responsibility of the person or entity initiating a

request for information to obtain the patient's authorization to disclose. For example, if an insurance company wants health care information about a certain patient, it has the responsibility of obtaining the patient's consent and giving it to the doctor. In the absence of the patient's explicit consent, no information should be provided.

- Written responses to inquiries must be made by the doctor. A staff member should never assume the responsibility of abstracting information from a patient's record and sending it to anyone without the doctor's supervision and signature on the document.
- Follow-up inquiries from insurance companies may be answered on the basis of the patient's original consent, provided the information requested does not exceed the authorization given by the patient. If it appears to exceed the authorization, the inquiry should not be answered until the patient's consent is provided.

In addition to keeping a constant vigil against the direct disclosure of confidential information, physicians and their staff should take certain precautions to avoid the inadvertent disclosure of information by doing the following:

- Keeping the appointment book, patient lists, patient files, and patient records out of public view.
- Positioning all computer terminals so that the screen cannot be seen by patients, messengers, or delivery persons. Patient information should never be left on an unattended screen; an automatic log-off, screen-saver, or fade-to-dim function should be installed.
- It is extremely important to establish a strict policy regarding personnel accessing only those records that they have a right to access. An employee who is discovered reading a patient record that he/she does not have a valid right to be reading is fired on

the spot by one large West Coast health management organization. The policy is well-known and strictly enforced.

- Asking another staff member to handle confidential information concerning a member of your family, a friend, or neighbor.
- Always conversing with patients in private regarding personal, health, or financial information.
- Discussing patients only with people who need the information and who are entitled to it.
- Never discussing patients outside the office or in front of other patients inside the office. Patient names should never be mentioned because the specialty of the doctor might disclose why the patient is being seen. Be aware of what is said in the hall or adjacent rooms. Patients in the reception area can frequently hear what is discussed behind that sliding window.
- Locating fax machines, printers, and copy machines in a secure area. When a fax is being received or when patient information is being printed or copied, the machine should never be left unattended.
- Always disposing of documents containing confidential patient information carefully—shredding or incinerating is best. A facility should have a signed nondisclosure statement with contracted recyclers.

COMPETENCY CHECK: THREE

7. **An optometry assistant receives a telephone call from Mr. Jones, who identifies himself as the Personnel Director of the Smith Industrial Company. He names a patient currently being treated by the doctor and says she is an employee of the Smith Company. He then says that the employee has called in sick for several days and that he is concerned about the extent of the employee's health problems. He asks the assistant to describe the employee's condition. How should the assistant respond?**

8. **List four precautions all staff should take to prevent the accidental disclosure of confidential patient information.**

CONFIDENTIALITY PROBLEMS

HIV Test Results

There is currently so much variation among state laws concerning the handling of the results of human immunodeficiency virus (HIV) testing that it is essential that each health care provider know what is required and what is allowed in his/her state. In some states, the results of HIV testing must be kept by the physician in a file that is separate from the patient health records. In other states, the results are kept in the patient's health record, but they must be kept in a sealed envelope. In some states, the results are included in the patient's health record and are available to other health care providers.

Fig. 4-B. Sample Informed Consent for HIV Antibody Test

I voluntarily give my consent to be tested for exposure to the Human Immunodeficiency Virus (HIV). HIV is the term used for the virus that is thought to cause AIDS. I understand that my blood will be drawn for the purpose of determining whether I have been exposed to this virus.

I understand that the exact meaning of an HIV antibody test result may not be clear in my case. A positive result does not mean that I will come down with AIDS. A negative result does not ensure that I do not have early HIV infection or that I cannot transmit the infection.

I understand that all reasonable efforts to provide confidentiality and/or anonymity to the extent provided by law will be made. However, I understand that the results of this test will be recorded in my medical record. As medical record information, these tests results will be regarded as confidential, and the Hospital will not disclose these test results to unauthorized third parties without my express written authorization. I understand, however, that confidentiality cannot be absolutely guaranteed, and that the results will be available to physicians and other health care professionals responsible for my care and treatment.

I understand that Illinois law requires that if this test result in combination with other data leads my physician to make a presumptive diagnosis of AIDS, then my case must be reported to the public health authorities and may be investigated by them.

I have been informed that if this test is positive a physician will provide counseling for follow-up care and for precautions against transmitting this infection.

I understand that if I refuse this test my exposure to the HIV will remain unknown. My ability to infect others with this virus will also remain unknown.

I warrant that I freely give my informed consent and that I have not been forced, coerced, or subjected to any constraint or inducement. I understand that I may withdraw this consent anytime prior to having my blood drawn.

I hereby give consent for the performance of the HIV antibody test.

I refuse consent for the performance of the HIV antibody test. I understand that this refusal may limit the clinical data available to my physician. However, this refusal will not affect my access to further care.

Signature _____   Date _____

Witness _____

Release of Information to Insurance Companies

When patients sign the waiver on an insurance claim form, they have authorized any physician, hospital, or other medical provider to release to the insurance company any information regarding their medical history, symptoms, treatment, examination results or diagnosis necessary to process the request. This opens the patients' files to any number of inquiries. Patients can limit this authorization by changing the release to read: ". . . to release to the insurance company the information regarding their medical history, symptoms, examination notes, or treatment necessary to process this request."

Health care providers can protect patient confidentiality by only providing the information requested instead of the entire record (e.g., if the request is concerned with an asthma condition, then the insurance company does not need earlier information regarding a sexually transmitted disease or an injury from being kicked by a horse). If the authorization is not dated, contact the patient in order to ascertain whether the request is to be honored. Health care providers should submit the minimum information possible within legal limits. They should also ask insurance carriers and others why they need the specific information, and verify the need with the patient.

The following is an example of what can happen if care is not taken in releasing a patient's records to a third party.

Skiing cross-country through a campus park one winter's day, University of Michigan graduate student Frank G. Palermo found himself perched atop a steep slope. Heart racing, he pushed off and sped downhill, only to come to a wrenching halt when his ski tips dug abruptly into the thin crust. The leather strap on his left ski pole snapped; so did his left thumb. Frank wound up at the University Hospital in Ann Arbor, where his doctors decided to operate. In preparation, they summoned his medical records from his family physician in Detroit.

According to Frank's file, he was a walking medical mine-field. "You appear to have had your gallbladder removed at age two," the doctors told him. "You've had kidney stones, a broken nose, and recently broke your leg." Frank was perplexed; except for the broken nose, the list of maladies was news to him. A phone call solved the mystery: It seems his family doctor had carelessly lumped his medical history in with those of his grandfather and cousin—both also named Frank G. Palermo.

Frank laughs about the snafu. But imagine another scenario, one that easily could have occurred had he not been able to set his medical records straight: Frank applies for individual health insurance and signs a standard waiver authorizing the insurer to obtain copies of his health files. With a supposed history of internal disorders and broken bones dating back to age two, he's clearly a bad risk and his application is rejected. Meanwhile—again acting on the waiver Frank signed—the insurance carrier feeds its findings to a computer bank that shares medical data with hundreds of other insurance companies.

Now, say that his grandfather or cousin had problems more controversial than gallstones or a broken leg—some psychiatric care, perhaps, or drug abuse, or (an increasingly daunting prospect today) a positive test for HIV . . . In addition to being rejected for insurance, Frank suffers a series of unaccountable setbacks. He applies for a postgraduate program, and is turned down. He sends out job applications, and is never called for an interview. And when Frank finally lands a second-rate job, his coworkers buzz about his "condition." He loses any chance of career advancement. Frank never suspects that it is his medical records—leaked to the world, containing mistakes he doesn't even know about—that have left his life in a shambles.

This has actually happened to people; a mistake that has impacted their lives for decades.[2]

Other Confidentiality Problems

Trouble can arise for a doctor when the patient has a terminal illness and either the patient or the family requests that the patient not be told of the true diagnosis and prognosis.

If a terminal diagnosis is kept from a patient, that patient may not put his/her "affairs in order." The patient may make decisions for the future that are inappropriate, given the prognosis. If neither the patient nor the family knows the diagnosis and prognosis because the patient instructed the doctor not to disclose the information, the family could sue for negligence after the death of the patient, unless the doctor has extremely good proof of the patient's instructions.

Treating famous patients (actors, actresses, politicians, music stars, and others) can be a real challenge to the maintenance of confidentiality. During the 1960 presidential campaign, John F. Kennedy's doctor kept his famous patient's record in a bank vault because his office was broken into and his records searched. When Marilyn Monroe was hospitalized in New York City's Lennox Hospital for a tubal repair, security was so effective that the media could not even learn the name of her doctor or the nature of her problem beyond "some kind of female problem."

Another question concerns the public's right to know if a government official has a serious health problem that might compromise that person's ability to function in that position. Legal opinions are inconclusive.

A problem for the doctor can stem from the presence of a socially unacceptable condition in a patient when the patient does not want the information entered on his/her record. This is particularly true in small communities where everyone knows or is related to everyone else, or in a situation in which the patient is well-known in the community.

A difficult confidentiality issue can occur in situations in which one partner in marriage (or domestic affairs) has a condition or situation that could affect the other partner, but to disclose would cause an interpersonal problem for the couple. There can be difficult situations, for example, in which it is crucial that a mother confide to the doctor that her husband is not her child's father.

SUMMARY

In this chapter you learned the importance of the confidentiality inherent in the physician-patient relationship—a principle dating back to Hippocrates in the fifth century B.C.—and the importance of the patient's right to privacy.

Confidentiality is protected not only because of ethical principle, but also by privileged communication statutes. Except under certain circumstances, only the patient—or the patient's family or guardian in the case of a minor or a mentally incompetent adult—can authorize disclosure of information about the patient's condition and treatment. Disclosure is allowed without the patient's consent if required by law, by subpoena or court order, to protect the health and welfare of the public, or if the disclosure is necessary to protect the well-being of the patient or another individual.

All members of the health care team are as ethically and legally bound to keep patient information confidential as is the doctor.

When you have finished reading this chapter, complete the corresponding chapter in your workbook and then go on to Chapter Five.

REFERENCES

1. Feste L. Guidelines for Faxing Patient Health Information. *Professional Medical Assistant.* May/June 1992;25:14.
2. Endicott J. Absolutely not Confidential. *Hippocrates.* March/April 1989:53-54.

5

Consent to Medical Treatment

With very few exceptions, mentally competent adults have the sole authority to decide what may be done to their bodies. Inherent in this authority is the right to give an informed consent to health care treatment. This chapter describes informed consent and the legal consequences of not obtaining proper informed consent. Also discussed are the questions of which persons actually have the authority to give consent, and which forms that consent may take.

OBJECTIVES

After studying this chapter, you will be able to:

1. Identify who must authorize treatment of a minor, an emancipated minor, and an adult under legal disability.
2. Contrast a fiduciary relationship with the normal buyer-seller relationship.
3. List four items of information that the doctrine of informed consent entitles each patient to have before authorizing medical treatment.
4. Identify the guidelines for disclosing information to patients and obtaining informed consent.
5. Explain the difference between the reasonable physician standard and the reasonable person standard with regard to determining negligence in informing patients of inherent risks.
6. Prepare a written consent form that incorporates the required information.

AUTHORITY TO TREAT

The right of an adult of sound mind to determine what can be done to his/her body is a long-recognized principle of law. Health care providers are legally obligated to obtain the patient's authorization before initiating treatment.

Adults

Authorization for treatment generally arises from valid consent of the patient. The patient must be of legal age; in most states, a person 18 years of age or older has the right to consent to medical treatment. A few states have set the age of consent at 19 or 21. If the patient is a minor, consent usually must be obtained from a parent or guardian.

The patient must also be mentally competent; therefore the patient must not be delirious, comatose, or under the influence of drugs or alcohol. If the patient is under legal disability, his/her spouse, parent, or court-appointed guardian must consent before treatment begins.

Historically, and for most conditions today, the parent or legal guardian of a minor child must consent before the minor receives treatment. The consent of one parent is usually sufficient. When parents are separated or divorced, the consent of the custodial parent is necessary.

> The aunt of a 15-year-old boy persuaded him to donate skin grafts for her child who had been severely burned. The boy lived with his mother, but she was not informed of the procedure or asked to consent. Complications during the procedure developed, and the boy was hospitalized for a long time. The mother sued for lack of parental consent. The court permitted the suit. (*Bonner v Moran*, 126 F.2d 121, Cal.D.C. 1941)

Exceptions to Consent for Minors

The general rule of requiring parental consent for the treatment of minors is subject to several exceptions.

- It is a widely-accepted judgment of the courts, and clarified by statute in many states, that in an emergency a doctor does not need to obtain parental permission before providing a minor with **emergency treatment.**

- If the parent of a minor needing nonemergency medical treatment refuses to consent out of neglect, ignorance, or religious belief, a **court order** authorizing the necessary treatment must be obtained before treatment begins.
- Some states have now established a **mature minor** rule that says that a minor can consent to any medical treatment if it is for himself/herself, if it is for his/her benefit, and if he/she understands the nature of the treatment and the nature of the procedure. Many states have passed legislation identifying minors, age of 14 (12 in California) and older, as statutory adults for the purposes of consent for medical treatment, confidentiality, privacy, and access to medical records. In other states, courts apply this rule in case law. Given this trend, doctors would be wise to obtain the consent of a minor approaching the age of majority, as well as that of the minor's parent. The AMA recommends obtaining the minor's consent after he/she reaches the age of 15.
- An **emancipated minor**, recognized by law in most states, is freed from many of the legal restrictions of minors and is considered capable of entering into legally binding contracts. A minor becomes emancipated when he/she:

1. joins the armed forces.
2. becomes a parent, whether married or not.
3. marries (separation, divorce, or death of spouse does not change the emancipated status).
4. lives separate from parents and earns an independent living, manages finances, and assumes an adult role.

   [California statutes allow minors 15 years or older who live apart from parents or legal guardians and who manage their own affairs to consent for routine medical care, regardless of their source of income.]

- Many states have passed laws permitting minors to be treated for **sexually transmitted disease** without parental consent. In the absence of a specific law to this effect, a doctor could treat a minor for sexually transmitted disease without parental consent on the grounds that the disease is a medical emergency. The AMA's official policy is that a doctor should never hesitate to treat a child with sexually transmitted disease if immediate treatment is required.
- Some states have passed legislation permitting doctors to provide minors with **contraceptives** without parental consent. Courts in other states have ruled that doctors may provide minors with contraceptives without parental consent on the grounds that a sexually active minor is a medical emergency.

    Any doctor personally opposed to providing minors with contraceptives has no obligation to do so. A doctor who provides a minor with contraceptives should:

    1. Inquire about the feasibility of parental consent, and encourage the minor to tell the parents.
    2. Carefully explain all potential side effects associated with the contraceptive and obtain the minor's written, informed consent.
    3. Keep detailed records, including an explanation of why the situation constituted a medical emergency requiring contraceptive treatment.

- Many states permit minors to obtain treatment related to **pregnancy** without parental consent, although some states exclude abortions.
- In every state by statute or case law doctors may treat minors for **drug addiction** without parental consent.

COMPETENCY CHECK: ONE

1. **True or false. Children and adults under legal disability will need someone else to consent for treatment.**

2. Whose consent should a surgeon obtain before per-
    forming a tonsillectomy on a 15-year-old with acutely
    infected tonsils?

Right to Refuse Treatment

A patient's right to authorize treatment includes the right to
terminate or refuse treatment. Terminally ill patients, in particular, are entitled to "die with dignity" and to prohibit the
use of extraordinary measures that postpone the inevitable.

FIDUCIARY RELATIONSHIPS

The relationship between highly-trained, service-oriented
professionals and the people seeking their services is fiduciary in nature, and is based on trust and confidence.

In the case of the doctor and patient, the fiduciary relationship is based on the patient's trust and confidence in the
doctor's knowledge and ability. This trust and confidence
obligates the doctor to act for the benefit of the patient. This
obligation includes the legal duty to voluntarily disclose all
information relevant to the treatment being proposed.

The doctor–patient relationship is but one example of a
fiduciary relationship. Other examples of fiduciary relationships are those between attorney and client, clergy and religious adherent, and trustor and trustee.

A fiduciary relationship contrasts with the normal
buyer-seller relationship in which an atmosphere of *caveat
emptor* "let the buyer beware" prevails. In the usual buyer-
seller relationship, the seller is not obligated (unless mandated by law) to voluntarily disclose any defects in the mer-
chandise he/she is selling; in a fiduciary relationship, the
professional party must disclose any reasonably foreseeable
dangers or risks inherent in the proposed service.

Forms of Consent

Implied Consent
For treatment of subsidiary medical problems routinely handled in a physician's office, the patient's actions imply

his/her consent. The patient has the prescription filled, accepts an injection, returns for follow-up appointments, etc. The same patient behaviors implying the establishment of a contract imply consent to treatment.

In most of these routine situations, where treatment of a minor problem is standardized throughout the medical profession and is of negligible risk, a patient's implied consent is sufficient for the legal protection of the physician. A possible exception to this would be a situation in which the physician recommends an experimental or unorthodox procedure. In such a situation, the patient's express consent should be obtained.

Express Consent

Express consent may be oral or written, but the written form is recommended whenever the proposed treatment involves surgery, experimental drugs, or high-risk procedures.

Written consent can reduce the possibility of misunderstanding between physician and patient. It can also facilitate proving what was mutually agreed to. Should a lawsuit develop, a written agreement can strengthen a patient's claim that the physician deviated from their agreement. Conversely, it can help the physician defend himself/herself against an unjustified claim.

Accurately remembering past oral agreements is difficult under the best of circumstances. When time, anxiety, and an unfortunate result intervene, an accurate recollection is often reduced to wishful thinking. An effective written statement executed at the time of the agreement can eradicate this problem.

Express written consent provides maximum protection for both patient and physician, but obtaining it is not always practical or necessary.

For treatment not involving major surgery or experimental or high-risk procedures, a patient's oral consent is often sufficient. A physician should, however, enter a note in the patient's chart that the proposed treatment was explained and orally agreed to by the patient. This note should be entered in the patient's medical record when the explanation was made and the consent given. The legal term for this type of entry is "written declaration."

The Office of the General Counsel of the American Medical Association has developed an array of standardized forms covering a board range of medical procedures for which express written consent is recommended. Two of these standardized forms are reproduced below in Figures 5-A and 5-B.

Note the steps taken in Figure 5-A, "Consent to Operation, Anesthetics, and Other Medical Services," to clarify what is to be done and to ensure that the patient is giving an informed consent.

Note also the following information pertaining to Figure 5-A:

- Item 2 should be modified if the physician's authority is to be limited.
- Item 3 is included because misunderstandings about anesthesia have resulted in many lawsuits.
- Item 4 directs the patient's attention to the importance of an informed consent.
- Item 5 deals with the guarantees and indicates that, under normal circumstances and in the absence of an agreement to the contrary, the physician does not guarantee the outcome of the procedure.
- Items 6-8 concern the patient's right to privacy and provide an opportunity to limit publicity.
- Item 9 is included because of special concerns in this area.
- Item 10 is for the legal protection of the patient and physician and is a way of ensuring the integrity of the consent.
- The direction to cross out any item(s) not applicable is a way of permitting modifications to a general form.

Figure 5-A. Sample Consent to Operation, Anesthetics, and Other Medical Services

Date _____ Time _____

A.M.
P.M.

1. I authorize the performance upon *(myself or name of patient)* of the following operation: *(state nature and extent of operation)* to be performed by or under the direction of Dr. _____.

2. I consent to the performance of operations and procedures in addition to or different from those now contemplated, whether or not arising from presently unforeseen conditions, which the above-named doctor or his/her associates or assistants may consider necessary or advisable in the course of the operation.

3. I consent to the administration of such anesthetics as may be considered necessary or advisable by the physician responsible for this service, with the exception of *(state "none," "spinal anesthesia," etc.)*.

4. The nature and purpose of the operation, possible alternative methods of treatment, the risks involved, the possible consequences, and the possibility of complications have been explained to me by Dr. _____ and by _____.

5. I acknowledge that no guarantee or assurance has been given by anyone as to the results that may be obtained.

6. I consent to the photographing or televising of the operations or procedures to be performed, including appropriate portions of my body, for medical, scientific, or educational purposes, provided my identity is not revealed by the pictures or by descriptive texts accompanying them.

7. For the purpose of advancing medical education, I consent to the admittance of observers to the operating room.

8. I consent to the disposal by hospital authorities of any tissues or body parts which may be removed.

9. I am aware that sterility may result from this operation. I know that a sterile person is incapable of becoming a parent.

10. I acknowledge that all blank spaces on this document have been either completed or crossed off prior to my signing.

(Cross out any paragraphs above which do not apply.)

Witness _____   Signature _____

(Patient or person authorized to consent for patient)

Source: Medicolegal Forms with Legal Analysis, *1973 ed, published by the American Medical Association. Reprinted with permission.*

Figure 5-B. Sample Authorization for Smallpox Vaccination

A.M.

Date _____ Time _____ P.M.

I (We) authorize Dr. _____ , the attending physician, to administer smallpox vaccination to _____ my (our) infant/self to provide immunization against smallpox.

It has been explained to me (us) that the United States Public Health Service "now believes that the risk of smallpox in the United States is so small that the practice of routine smallpox vaccination is no longer indicated in this country." It has further been explained that the Public Health Service has published a statement that the risk of complications resulting from vaccination is greater than the probability of contracting the disease unless travel to and from a country where smallpox is endemic is planned, or unless contact with patients who have the disease is possible.

Dr. _____ has also explained that the vaccination cannot be administered if (I) my (our) child has eczema or other forms of chronic dermatitis or has household contacts with these conditions or has an altered immune state because of diseases such as _____ or therapy (or pregnancy if the recipient is a female of child-bearing age) and I (we) have assured him/her that none of these conditions exist.

I (We) voluntarily consent to the administration of the small-pox vaccination and release Dr. _____ from liability for any results that may occur.

Witness _____   Signed _____

(Patient or person(s) autho-
rized to consent for patient)

Source: Medicolegal Forms with Legal Analysis, *1973 ed, published by the American Medical Association. Reprinted with permission.*

The use of a broad or "blanket" consent form—one that does not specify the procedure to be performed, but grants total authority to a physician—is generally discouraged. When a defendant–physician has exhibited a blanket form in court as justification for performing a certain procedure, some courts have construed the form to cover only those procedures to which the patient had orally agreed. In other words, the written consent is virtually disregarded, and it becomes a matter of which party's oral testimony the judge or jury believes.

> A woman consented orally to an appendectomy. The surgeon removed her appendix and, as a precautionary measure, performed a total hysterectomy. The patient sued for unauthorized surgery. In his defense the physician produced the following form that had been signed by the patient:

AUTHORITY TO OPERATE

Date 3/17/58

I hereby authorize the Physician or Physicians in charge to administer such treatment and the surgeon to have administered such anesthetics as found necessary to perform this operation which is advisable in the treatment of this patient.

Witness ___JLT___   Signed _Dolly Rogers_

In commenting on this form, the court said: "We think the so-called authorization is so ambiguous as to be almost completely worthless, and, certainly, since it fails to designate the nature of the operation authorized and for which consent was given, it can have no possible weight under the factual circumstances of the instant case."

This noteworthy case, however, was not resolved on this issue alone. Also taken into consideration and given considerable weight was the fact that the patient had been treated by the physician-defendant for her inability to conceive. Hence, the physician knew of her desire to have children, but proceeded anyway—and in the absence of an emergency—to eliminate any possibility of the patient bearing children. The court found for the plaintiff. (*Rogers v Lumbermens Mutual Casualty*, 119 So.2d 649, La. 1960)

Informed Consent

The fiduciary nature of the doctor–patient relationship, coupled with the long-held axiom that an adult of "sound mind has the right to determine what shall be done with his/her own body,"[1] obligates doctors to obtain a patient's informed consent before beginning medical treatment. This consent must develop from the patient's understanding of the:

- General nature of the proposed care and the results it might predictably have on the patient's body.
- Normal risks and hazards inherent in the proposed treatment and the likelihood of each risk occurring.
- Side effects or complications known normally to occur, and their severity and permanence.
- Alternative treatments (including no treatment) and the probable outcome of each.

Only when the consent stems from an understanding of the foregoing is the patient able to give an informed consent. To paraphrase a statement made by one court, every person of sound mind is entitled to say whether he/she gets cut, by whom he/she gets cut, and where he/she gets cut. For this to be a meaningful decision, the patient must know the serious risks inherent in the contemplated procedure and must know the alternatives available.

COMPETENCY CHECK: TWO

3. With regard to disclosing information, what does the fiduciary nature of the doctor-patient relationship obligate doctors to do?

4. What two legal principles combine to obligate a doctor to obtain a patient's informed consent prior to medical treatment?

5. List four general aspects the patient must understand before it can be said that the patient's consent is truly informed.

Guidelines Concerning Disclosures

When explaining a proposed treatment and its inherent risks, doctors must exercise good medical judgment and proceed in a way that promotes the patient's genuine understanding of the explanation.

A comprehensive list of information that should be given every patient is impossible because each patient requires a tailor-made explanation, but the following principles should guide doctors:

- The greater the risk involved—with regard to the likelihood of occurrence, permanence, or severity—the greater the doctor's obligation of disclosure. The law does not require or expect doctors to report every side effect or bad result that has ever been reported in the medical literature, nor does it expect doctors to report commonly known risks, such as infections after surgery. Doctors are expected to inform patients of any life-threatening risks and of those risks known to occur with some regularity under normal circumstances.
- Alternative treatments should be disclosed that are recommended by at least a respectable number of reasonable doctors. If the patient selects an alternative treatment, the doctor is not obligated to provide it, but should suggest a reputable doctor who might.

A doctor recommended an operation to a patient with prostate problems that would leave the patient sterile. The doctor did not tell the patient of this side effect, nor did he tell him of an alternative procedure that carried a higher risk of infection but would not necessarily result in sterility. The patient agreed to the operation recommended by the doctor. He discovered later that he was sterile and sued the doctor. The suit was decided in the patient's favor, and the court said that, in the absence of an emergency, the patient was entitled to know all of the options and to select the one he preferred. (*Bang v Charles T. Miller Hospital*, 88 N.W.2d 186, Min. 1958)

- If the proposed treatment is unorthodox or experimental, the patient should be so informed and also notified that all risks may not be known.
- If a general practitioner offers service customarily provided by a specialist, the patient should be told the usual practice and given the option of a referral.
- Reasonable measures should be taken to ensure the patient's understanding of the doctor's explanation. The doctor should use terms understandable and meaningful to each individual patient. Several lawsuits have resulted from a patient's ignorance of the medical terms used to describe a proposed treatment. A valid consent never stems from ignorance.

A patient consented to a laminectomy that left him paralyzed. It was shown in the ensuing lawsuit that the patient never understood the term "laminectomy" or what the procedure entailed. Further, there was no evidence that the defendant surgeon warned him of any risks. The court found in favor of the patient on the grounds of no informed consent. (*Gray v Grunnagle*, 223 A.2d 663, Pa. 1966)

An atmosphere of open communication between doctor and patient should be fostered. Allied health professionals can help to create and maintain a candid and relaxed atmosphere. Their assistance in this area can be invaluable to the medical practice. Some patients find it easier to express their concerns to allied health personnel than to doctors. In addition to listening carefully and respectfully, these personnel should urge patients to discuss their concerns directly with the doctor. If a patient refuses to do so, the allied health professionals should promptly relay the patient's concerns.
- Including the patient's spouse in a discussion of proposed treatment is often recommended for the sake of both the patient and doctor. Of course, spousal consent to therapeutic treatment is never required, and if the patient objects to the presence of any third party, such wishes must be honored.

HIV Testing

The principle of informed consent is basically valid in the case of HIV testing, although there have been conflicting court opinions and legislation in many states that have modified this principle. The following excerpt discussing a 1993 Florida statute and its application is instructive:

An HIV test may not be administered without uncoerced informed consent. The subject must be told that the test and result will be maintained as protected confidential information. Consent need not be written, but the physician must document in the patient's health record that the test was explained and consent obtained. If the subject is a minor, incompetent, or incapable of informed judgment, consent must be obtained from the legal guardian.

The statute allows an exception for examination and treatment of sexually transmitted diseases for any minor. If a parent or guardian accompanies the minor, testing would require consent of the parent or guardian. If the minor seeks testing without their knowledge, consent is not a prerequisite and informing the parents or guardian is prohibited.

Informed consent is not required for testing a person who has been convicted of prostitution or procuring the services of prostitution. HIV testing by a medical examiner does not require consent. Exceptions also exist for cornea removal or enucleation. If a voluntarily obtained or court ordered blood sample, drawn for other purposes, already exists for a defendant in a sexual battery prosecution, the victim may request that the blood sample be tested for HIV without the defendant's informed consent.

If the parent of a hospitalized infant cannot be found after a reasonable attempt, informed consent is not required to perform an HIV test for a medical diagnosis necessary to appropriate care.

In bona fide medical emergencies, when the patient is unable to consent, an HIV test necessary to medical diagnosis for emergency care may be performed without informed consent. When an HIV test is necessary for medical diagnosis of an acute illness, yet seeking informed consent would be detrimental to the patient, the test may be performed without informed consent.

If medical personnel sustain significant exposure to a person of unknown HIV status, an already existing blood sample may be tested for HIV, but only after the patient has been provided an opportunity to "consent."[2]

Doctrine of Professional Discretion

A doctor may justifiably withhold information from a patient in some cases. When a patient appears emotionally unstable or unduly anxious, a doctor may withhold information for therapeutic reasons, particularly if the risks are quite improbable and not serious. Known risks and alternative treatments should, however, be explained to the patient's spouse or next of kin. Furthermore, high-risk treatment, such as chemotherapy, electroshock therapy, and radiation therapy, should always be explained to the patient regardless of how the information might affect his/her morale.

If a patient expressly says he/she does not want to know about the proposed treatment or the risks involved, the doctor need not force the patient to listen. For legal protection, the doctor should ask the patient to sign a statement waiving the right to the information. In addition, the doctor should explain the procedure and its risks to the patient's spouse or next of kin.

Extending Operations

The doctrine of informed consent poses special concerns for surgeons. Occasionally, they discover an unexpected condition during surgery that requires a treatment different from that which the patient authorized.

When the unanticipated condition constitutes an emergency—defined as an immediate threat to the patient's health—the surgeon may extend the procedure to remove the threat. In such a case, the legal principle would be that the patient's consent is implied.

A doctor performed surgery for an anticipated tubal pregnancy. After surgery began, the doctor realized the patient had a normal pregnancy but an acutely infected appendix, which he removed. The patient's husband refused to pay the surgeon on the grounds that an appendectomy was not consented to. The court ruled in favor of the doctor and noted that the infected appendix constituted an emergency and its removal was good medical practice. (*Barnett v Bachrach*, 34 A.2d 626, D.C. 1943)

When the situation is not a true emergency, but good surgical practice, and the patient's best interests suggest an extension, many courts will not penalize a doctor for extending a procedure simply because it was not specifically authorized. According to the court in *Barnett v. Bachrach*, "The law does not insist that a surgeon shall perform every operation according to plans and specifications approved in advance by the patient and carefully tucked away in his office safe for courtroom purposes."[3]

Extending an operation in the absence of a genuine emergency is not without legal risk to the surgeon. A prudent surgeon takes several steps to ensure that he/she is acting in the patient's best interests and, at the same time, is minimizing liability.

- He/she makes sure the consent form executed by the patient includes a statement authorizing him/her to extend the operation if necessary.
- The surgeon explains the situation and obtains the consent of the spouse or next of kin, if available, on behalf of the patient.

  While performing an appendectomy on a 20-year-old girl, a surgeon noted that her fallopian tubes were seriously infected. He decided to remove them. He did not consult the girl's stepmother beforehand, although he knew she was in the hospital. The surgeon was sued for unauthorized treatment and found liable. The situation did not constitute an emergency, and the girl's problem could have been resolved in less drastic ways. (*Tabor v Scobee*, 254 S.W.2d 474, Ky. 1952)

- Whenever abdominal or pelvic surgery is contemplated that could involve the patient's sexual or reproductive functions, the surgeon and the patient should agree before surgery how the surgeon will proceed if an extension of surgery affecting either of these functions becomes necessary.

Exceptions to the Necessity of Consent

Situations in which consent for treatment is not required include those in which:

- Consent is assumed (e.g., in any life- or limb-threatening emergency).
- The law requires a certain treatment (e.g., vaccinations for school entry).
- A court order has been issued. A typical situation resulting in a court order is a parent refusing life-saving treatment for a minor child.

COMPETENCY CHECK: THREE

6. The doctor's obligation to disclose a risk increases in proportion to what?

7. Describe three situations in which a doctor would not be obligated to obtain a patient's informed consent prior to initiating treatment.

8. A doctor recommends an experimental drug. In addition to the known risks, what must the physician tell the patient?

9. Why does the doctrine of informed consent pose special concerns for surgeons?

LEGAL CONSEQUENCES

Assault and Battery

A doctor who treats a patient without permission may be sued for assault and battery.

No matter how ill the patient or how effective a proposed treatment, a patient has the right to refuse it. Forcing a patient to accept treatment or imposing it in any way without consent constitutes assault and battery.

A gynecologist performed an exploratory laparotomy and oophorectomy on a patient, who was a registered nurse. She experienced serious postoperative complications and subsequently sued the gynecologist for negligence and battery. The battery complaint was based on her allegation that she clearly told the gynecologist she wanted a particular surgeon present during the operation and had made arrangements for the surgeon to be there. She testified that the morning of the operation she told the gynecologist she did not want to be anesthetized until the surgeon arrived, but the gynecologist proceeded in the surgeon's absence. The jury ruled that the negligence charge was unfounded but the battery charge was not. It awarded the patient $75,000. On appeal, the Supreme Court of Virginia upheld the verdict and said that because the doctor–patient relationship is a consensual one, surgery without proper authorization is a battery. It added that a patient has the right to withdraw consent if done in clear terms and at an opportune time. (*Pugsley v Privette*, 263 S.E.2d 69 Va. 1980)

Negligence

A doctor who obtains a patient's consent but does not properly explain risks inherent in the proposed treatment may be sued on the grounds of professional negligence. The plaintiff's complaint is not that the doctor failed to perform the procedure properly, but that the doctor failed to *explain* it properly. Cases alleging negligence are much more common than those alleging assault and battery.

To have a legitimate negligence case, the plaintiff-patient must be able to show each of the following:

- That he/she suffered the possible consequence the doctor failed to explain or explain properly. (Merely learning after the procedure has been performed that information was withheld would not in and of itself justify a claim.)
- That if he/she had known of the risk, he/she would have refused the treatment.
- That it was the practice of other doctors in the same or similar community, in the same or similar circumstances, to disclose the risk. Expert medical testimony will be required to prove this claim.

A thyroidectomy was performed on a patient, and the procedure damaged the patient's laryngeal nerve. The patient sued the doctor on the grounds that he was negligent in not disclosing the risk. Expert medical testimony showed that disclosing this risk was not the community practice. The doctor-defendant was, therefore, not liable for failing to inform the patient. (*Di Fillipo v Preston*, 173 A.2d 333, Del. 1961)

A trend, however, is developing that permits laymen to determine what must be disclosed. Referred to as the Canterbury Rule, this new theory says that, since the patient has the sole right to decide whether to have treatment, the right to information should not be determined by the medical profession. According to this theory, the patient is entitled to be informed of all *material* risks. A material risk is one a "reasonable person" would consider significant.

In explaining the Canterbury Rule, the Supreme Court of Wisconsin said:

The right of the patient and the duty of the doctor are standards recognized and circumscribed by the law and are not entirely dependent upon the customs of a profession. The need of a particular patient for competent expert information should not necessarily be limited to a self-created custom of the profession. The disclosures which would be made by doctors of good standing, under the same or similar circumstances, are certainly relevant and material and we surmise would be adequate to fulfill the doctor's duty of disclosure in most instances. However, the duty to disclose or inform cannot be summarily limited to a professional standard that may be nonexistent or inadequate to meet the informational needs of a patient.[4]

Courts in some states have refused to adopt the Canterbury Rule and continue to determine negligence in informing patients by the same standard used to determine negligence in other areas (i.e., the standard of care provided by other reasonable physicians).

In refusing the Canterbury Rule, one court said it would further increase the number of suits against physicians, which is already too high.[5] Nevertheless, the trend seems to be toward measuring a physician's disclosure of risks against what a reasonable person would consider material.

10. In most lawsuits against doctors that are based on the complaint of assault and battery, what do the plaintiffs allege that the doctor-defendants did not do?

11. Explain the difference between the "reasonable physician" standard and the "reasonable person" standard with regard to determining whether a physician was negligent in explaining to a patient the proposed treatment.

12. Define a *material* risk.

SUMMARY

The fiduciary relationship between physician and patient is based on trust and confidence. The nature of the relationship obligates the physician to act for the benefit of the patient. Included in this obligation is the physician's duty to voluntarily inform the patient of all relevant information concerning the treatment being offered, including potential hazards and risks. This duty and the long-recognized legal principle that a mentally competent adult has control over his/her own body require a physician to obtain the patient's informed consent before beginning medical treatment.

Consent must develop from the patient's understanding of the:

- General nature of the treatment and any consequences involved.
- Normal risks and hazards inherent in the treatment.
- Side effects or complications that may occur.
- Alternative treatments.

Although information is the basis of informed consent, there are some situations in which withholding information may be justifiable—for example, when a patient appears emotionally unstable or unduly anxious, particularly if the risks are quite improbable and not serious. Known risks and alternative treatments should, however, be explained to the patient's spouse or next of kin.

There are also exceptions to the necessity for obtaining consent. This is true when:

- Consent is assumed—e.g., in a life-threatening emergency.
- The law requires a certain treatment—e.g., vaccinations for school children.
- A court order has been issued.

Legal consequences for treating a patient without proper informed consent include charges of assault and battery and negligence. Treating a patient without permission is grounds for an assault and battery charge. If a physician obtains the patient's consent but neglects to properly explain the risks inherent in the procedure, he/she may be vulnerable to a negligence charge.

In the matter of consent, the question also arises as to who has the authority to give consent. In general, the mentally competent adult gives consent for his/her own treatment, while the parent or legal guardian gives consent for the treatment of a minor, unless he/she is an emancipated minor—one living independently and physically apart from parents.

There are two forms of consent—implied and express. Implied consent is reflected in the patient's actions—such as accepting an injection or having a prescription filled. Express consent is an oral or written acceptance of the treatment. While express consent may be either oral or written, the written form is recommended whenever the proposed treatment involves surgery, experimental drugs or procedures, or high-risk diagnostic or treatment procedures.

When you have finished reading this chapter, complete the corresponding chapter in your workbook and then go on to Chapter Six.

REFERENCES

1. Schloendorff v Society of New York Hospital, 105 N.E. 92, 93 (N.Y. Ct. App. 1914).
2. Allen WL. HIV Testin. *J. Florida MA* January 1994;81:35-36.

3. Barnett v Bachrach, 34 A2d 626, 629 (D.C. Mun. Ct. App. 1943).
4. Scaria v St. Paul Fire and Marine Insurance Co., 227 N.W.2d 647, 653 (Wis. 1975).
5. Bly v Rhoads, 222 S.E.2d 783, 787 (Va. 1976).

6

Negligence

The duty to provide reasonable care is one of the many obligations the health care professional owes his/her patients. Failure to provide it may result in the health care professional being found liable for professional negligence. The tort of negligence, professional negligence suits, and the doctrine of *respondeat superior* are the primary subjects of this chapter.

OBJECTIVES

After studying this chapter's contents, you will be able to:

1. Define and give examples of the terms reasonable doctor, reasonable allied health professional, reasonable care, and standard of care.
2. Explain the locality rule and its application to current day lawsuits.
3. List and explain the three major points the plaintiff in a professional negligence suit has to prove to be successful.
4. State the most significant differences between the ordinary professional negligence suit and one based on the doctrine of *res ipsa loquitur*.
5. Explain the purpose of damages in a civil suit and the three types of damages recognized by the legal system.
6. Define the doctrine of *respondeat superior* and explain how it applies to the doctor-employer/allied health professional relationship.
7. Define and give examples of the following terms: tort, course and scope of employment, vicarious liability, wrongful death, expert witness, and ordinary witness.

THE TORT OF NEGLIGENCE

A *tort* is a civil wrong for which the wrongdoer is liable to the wronged party for damages. Failing to act with reasonable care constitutes the tort of negligence. A legal definition of negligence is the "omission to do something which a reasonable person guided by those ordinary considerations which ordinarily regulate human affairs would do, or the doing of something which a reasonable and prudent person would not do."[1]

In describing this reasonable and prudent person, A. P. Herbert, a famous English attorney, wrote: "This excellent but odious character stands like a monument in our Courts of Justice vainly appealing to his fellow citizens to order their lives after his own example."[2]

Lawsuits alleging either personal negligence or professional negligence are governed by similar principles of tort law. There is an important difference, however, when these principles are applied to individual cases. That difference is the standard to which the defendants are held. In personal negligence cases, the defendant is held to the "reasonable person" standard. In professional negligence cases, the defendant is held to the "reasonable member of the profession" standard. In a suit against an architect, the standard is the reasonable architect; in a suit against an attorney, the standard is the reasonable attorney; in a suit against a physician, the standard is the reasonable physician.

THE STANDARD OF MEDICAL CARE

Determining a "reasonable" physician and "reasonable" medical care are legal issues resolved years ago, and most courts concur with the standards expressed in the following statement:

> The doctor is required to possess that degree of knowledge and skill, and to exercise that degree of care, judgment, and skill, which other doctors of good standing of the same school or system of practice usually exercise in the same or similar localities under like or similar circumstances.

Let's study the important phrases composing this statement, together with cases that illustrate the principles expressed:

The doctor is required to possess that degree of knowledge and skill . . .

These words express the need for the doctor to have the proper amount of education and experience. While this is usually interpreted to mean medical education and training, the statement has also been interpreted to mean the ability to communicate with each patient and to have access to necessary equipment. The physician who does not have the necessary knowledge, skill, or equipment must refer the patient to someone who does. This statement also obligates a physician to refer a patient to a specialist when it is apparent that the problem requires a specialist's skill and knowledge.

A general surgeon performed a hysterectomy in a hospital with limited facilities. The next day the surgeon realized that the patient had peritonitis but delayed for six days having her transferred to a better hospital and to the care of a trained specialist. After the transfer was made, the specialist removed a gangrenous intestine, but the patient died from complications due to the infection. The surgeon who performed the hysterectomy was liable because he did not send the patient to the specialist as soon as her condition required. (*Richardson v Holmes,* 525 S.W.2d 293, Tex. 1975)

A doctor's obligation to possess knowledge and skill certainly includes the duty to keep abreast of medical advancements in his/her field.

A patient's eyesight was permanently damaged by medication prescribed by her doctor. This doctor had not read any of numerous articles in medical journals describing the side effects of the prescribed medication, and he was found negligent for not keeping up to date. (*Reed v Church,* 8 S.E.2d 285, Va. 1940)

. . . to exercise that degree of care, judgment, and skill . . .

This phrase requires doctors to diligently apply their knowledge and skill; to know what to do and then to do it.

In addition to correctly performing medical procedures, doctors must see their patients as often as necessary and must be available to them. Recall the discussion in Chapter Three about the fact that the doctor who fails to see his/her patient often enough may be sued for abandonment or negligence. When the action is deliberate avoidance or when it is an improper termination of the contract, the suit would probably be based on a theory of abandonment. When a doctor makes an error in judgment concerning the necessity of seeing a patient, the grounds of the suit would probably be negligence.

Allied health professionals can help doctors fulfill their obligations to see their patients often enough by properly handling telephone calls and office visits, by knowing how to reach their doctor-employers quickly, and by making sure the telephone is covered by a qualified person or answering service when the office is closed.

The broad obligation to exercise due care, judgment, and skill also includes the specific obligations to give clear instructions to patients or their representatives, to warn patients about drug actions and possible effects, and to see that patients are properly cared for in the doctor's absence.

> A physician performed a tonsillectomy in his office early one morning. About 4:00 p.m., the patient's friend arrived to take her home. The friend saw that the patient was covered with blood and inquired into her well-being. The physician said only that she was OK and told the friend to take her home. He gave no further instructions and asked the friend no further questions. The patient was taken home and put to bed, and her friend then left for her own home. The patient's husband arrived a couple of hours later and discovered that his wife had bled to death. He sued the physician. The court said that as a general rule, due care requires physicians to give proper instructions and to be sure a person taking care of a patient is qualified. With regard to this particular case, the court said the patient should never have been released to the care of an untrained neighbor. The physician was found liable. (*Bateman v Rosenberg*, 525 S.W.2d 753, Mo. 1975)

In several lawsuits, doctors have been found negligent for not warning patients that prescribed medicine would make them drowsy and therefore unable to operate a vehicle properly. These suits have been filed not only by patients injured in accidents caused by their own drowsiness, but also by persons injured by drowsy patients. Doctors must warn patients to avoid operating an automobile or any dangerous equipment whenever their condition or treatment might impair their ability to do so. Warning patients about aspects of their conduct or treatment that pose a threat to the well-being of others is another situation in which the doctor's responsibilities extend beyond his/her patients. Recall from Chapter Four that, in certain instances, doctors must warn third parties about a patient's violent threats.

> A patient sought treatment from a physician for the relief of seizures. The physician agreed to treat the patient but did not make an immediate diagnosis; nor did he advise the patient to stop driving until the seizures were under control. A few days later the patient had a seizure while driving his car, lost control of it, and struck a pedestrian. The court permitted the pedestrian to sue the physician, and the pedestrian was awarded damages. (*Freese v Lemmon*, 210 N.W.2d 576, Iowa 1973)

. . . which other doctors of good standing of the same school or system of practice usually exercise in the same or similar localities under like or similar circumstances.

This clause is important because it establishes the standard to which a defendant-doctor will be held—the standard of care practiced by his/her peers. A doctor is legally obligated to provide *average* care when compared to other doctors:

. . . of the same school or system of practice . . .

"Same school" means schools founded on the same scientific theories and teaching the same or similar subject matter of equivalent depth and duration. In essence, physicians are compared to physicians, not podiatrists, dentists, or chiropractors. Likewise, podiatrists are compared to podiatrists, not osteopaths, pharmacists, or optometrists.

A patient sued a podiatrist and two physicians for negligence. The plaintiff's expert witness was a general surgeon, who was asked the standard of care for podiatrists. Defense counsel for the podiatrist objected on the grounds that a physician isn't qualified to discuss the standard of care for podiatrists; the court sustained the objection, noting that, since podiatry was different from general surgery, the surgeon was not qualified to discuss the standard of care. (*Darby v Cohen*, 421 N.Y.S.2d 337, S.C. 1979)

Most courts further limit the basis of comparison to like specialists. A family physician's knowledge, judgment, and skill are compared to that of other family physicians. Similarly, internists are compared to internists, surgeons to surgeons, dermatologists to dermatologists, etc.

> ... *in the same or similar localities under like or similar circumstances.*

In the past, this "locality rule" was applied to all suits alleging professional negligence. Under this rule, the prevailing medical practices of doctors within the defendant's community (or a similar community) were considered the norm or standard of care to which the defendant-doctor was held. The locality rule was strictly applied years ago because it was thought unfair to hold a doctor who practiced in a rural community unable to support a modern facility or variety of specialists to the same standard as a city colleague who had the advantages of access to an elaborate medical center and to many specialists.

Today, however, the locality rule no longer is applied automatically. In fact, it is usually dispensed with in lawsuits involving specialists, who are normally held to the standard of care practiced nationally.

A pediatrician did not perform a phenylketonuria test on a newborn. The baby had the disease and was permanently impaired by the delayed diagnosis. The pediatrician showed that the test was not usually done in the community's hospitals, but the parents showed it was routinely done throughout the country. The court held the pediatrician to the national standard and found him negligent. (*Naccarato v Grob*, 180 N.W.2d 788, Mich. 1970)

A patient sued a clinic surgeon for negligence in removing her breasts. The trial judge refused to permit the plaintiff's expert witness—a board certified surgeon—to testify because he was not familiar with the standard of care in the plaintiff's community. The appellate court upheld the trial judge's decision, but the state supreme court overruled the decision. It said that the witness was a specialist, as evidenced by his board certification, and that the standard of care for a specialist was a national standard. Therefore, the local standard was the same as the national one, with which the plaintiff's expert was familiar. A new trial was ordered. (*Francisco v Parchment Medical Clinic*, 285 N.W.2d 39, Mich. 1979.)

Even when the locality rule is applied, many courts no longer consider the prevailing community standard of paramount importance. "In most jurisdictions today, the local standard of practice is considered only one factor presented for the jury's determination and is not in and of itself determinative of the presence or absence of negligence."[3]

In summary, a doctor provides patients with reasonable care when treating patients with the same degree of knowledge, skill, and care that peers would provide under the same or similar circumstances. This principle is, however, easier to state than it is to apply, because it suggests that a standard or routine way of treating all medical problems exists or that good medicine can be provided by following the same recipe that other physicians use.

There are standardized treatments for some problems, and when the treatment is routine, universally practiced, and usually effective, a doctor would be well-advised to employ it. For many problems, however, the treatment is not routine, and even experts disagree on the best procedure. Legally, doctors might be safer to use a treatment recommended by the majority of their peers, but the law does not presume a doctor negligent for using a different treatment, provided it is accepted by a "respectable minority" of doctors and the patient gives an informed consent.

A patient underwent hip surgery, and her sciatic nerve was damaged in the process. The patient sued the surgeon and presented an expert witness who stated there were two ways of performing the surgery: that which the defendant used and that which the expert preferred because he believed it was less likely to cause nerve damage. The court dismissed the plaintiff's case, noting that a difference of opinion is not evidence of negligence. The court said, "Differences of opinion are consistent with the exercising of due care or even the highest degree of care." (*Kortus v Jensen*, 237 N.W.2d 845, Neb. 1976)

THE STANDARD OF CARE FOR ALLIED HEALTH PROFESSIONALS

The principle of determining reasonable care in accordance with how reputable members of the same profession act applies to negligence suits against any health care professional. A registered nurse would be held to the standard of reasonable registered nurses; a radiologic technologist would be held to the standard practiced by other reasonable radiologic technologists. A medical assistant would be held to the standard practiced by other reasonable medical assistants in the same or similar circumstances.

Under the principle of comparing like practitioners, the courts have ruled that when a nondoctor attempts to practice medicine, or performs any act that constitutes the practice of medicine, the nondoctor will be held to the standard of care applicable to doctors.

A drugless healer treated a patient who showed symptoms of appendicitis with enemas, laxatives, hot and cold packs, and electric massage. Despite a request from the patient's wife to call a physician, the healer refused. The wife contacted a surgeon, but peritonitis had occurred by the time the patient was hospitalized, and he died. The court ruled that once the healer "left the confines of his limited practice," he was obligated to meet the due care requirements of standard medical treatment. He was liable for not meeting them. (*Kelly v Carroll*, 219 P.2d 79, Wa. 1950)

COMPETENCY CHECK: ONE

1. Define a tort.

2. Define negligence.

3. Define professional negligence and give an example.

4. A doctor owes his/her patient the standard of care. Define "standard of care."

5. How does the locality rule influence the standard of care?

PROFESSIONAL NEGLIGENCE SUITS

The vast majority of lawsuits against health care professionals are based on the allegation of professional negligence. To prevail in this type of suit, the plaintiff must prove that the health care professional: (1) owed the patient the standard of care; (2) was negligent; and (3) that the negligence was the proximate cause of the patient's injuries.

Obligation for the Standard of Care

Following is a more detailed explanation of the plaintiff's task in proving the allegations.

Since this obligation is established when the doctor–patient relationship is established, the plaintiff must simply show the existence of the doctor–patient relationship. Ordinarily this is not difficult for the plaintiff to prove unless several defendants are named in the suit. When this happens, the plaintiff must show that a duty was owed him/her by each defendant.

Suppose, for example, a patient who was referred to a specialist by a family doctor attempts to hold both doctors liable for an injury sustained while under the care of the specialist. Assuming due care was used by the family doctor in making the referral, the family doctor would not be responsible for an injury caused by the specialist.

The referral served to terminate the relationship between the family doctor and patient, at least with regard to the problem for which the patient was referred. If, however, the referring doctor continued to care for the patient, he/she may or may not be jointly liable with the specialist. Liability would depend on the circumstances surrounding the case.

Negligence of the Doctor

The plaintiff will have to show that the doctor either did something that a reasonable doctor would not have done, or failed to do something that a reasonable doctor would have done. Notice that *the test is not whether the diagnosis was correct or the treatment effective, but whether the doctor met the standard of care.*

> A 32-year old woman was diagnosed with an enlarged fibroid in the uterus and probable cervical stenosis. Two pregnancy tests were negative. Just after making the incision for a hysterectomy, the surgeon discovered the patient was pregnant and terminated the surgery. The patient lost the baby and sued the surgeon for negligence. The court found in favor of the physician because due care was used in making the diagnosis. (*Hoglin v Brown*, 481 P.2d 458, Wa. 1971)

Negligence as the Proximate Cause of Injury

The plaintiff must prove that the doctor's negligence injured the patient. This point, known as proximate cause, requires that the plaintiff show a *direct* cause-and-effect relationship between the negligent act and the injury for which the plaintiff is claiming damages. No matter how negligent a doctor may have been, damages will not be awarded unless the negligence directly caused harm.

A diagnostic error or a delayed diagnosis due to negligence is not sufficient cause for a lawsuit, unless the plaintiff can demonstrate that the error or delay injured the patient.

> A patient's cervical vertebra was fractured in an automobile accident, but the fracture was not discovered for two months. The patient sued the physician for delayed diagnosis. Defense expert witnesses successfully showed that the treatment would have been the same if the diagnosis had been made immediately. The court held that, since the delay did not worsen the patient's condition or make a difference in the treatment, proximate cause was not established. (*Rudick v Prinerville Memorial Hospital*, 319 F.2d 764, CCA 9, 1963)

Preponderance of Evidence

The plaintiff must prove all three of the foregoing points by a "preponderance of evidence." He/she need not show the defendant culpable beyond a reasonable doubt—the requirement in a criminal case. In a civil case, the plaintiff's evidence must simply be more convincing to the jury or judge than the defendant's evidence. If the evidence on both sides is equal in merit, the decision must be for the defendant.

COMPETENCY CHECK: TWO

6. True or False: To win the suit, the plaintiff in a professional negligence suit must show only that the defendant did not provide the patient with reasonable care.

7. True or False: Proximate cause may be defined as the degree to which the plaintiff must prove his/her case.

8. True or False: The doctor's duty to provide a patient with reasonable care is established with the formation of the doctor–patient relationship.

9. True or False: The plaintiff in a civil suit must show the defendant culpable beyond a shadow of a doubt.

Expert Medical Testimony

A judge or jury of lay persons cannot normally be expected to know the standard of medical care to determine whether it was met, or to identify the existence of proximate cause. To show these points, the plaintiff must obtain and rely on testimony from one or more expert medical witnesses.

The status of "expert witness" is conferred upon those people who, through education and/or experience, have knowledge of matters that people lacking that education or experience do not have. In contrast to an "ordinary witness" who may testify only to facts known firsthand, an expert witness may testify to known and assumed facts, give an opinion, and answer hypothetical questions.

In virtually all professional negligence suits against doctors, expert medical testimony may be given only by another doctor. If the case involves a specialist, usually the expert must be from the same specialty as the defendant or from a closely related one. If a court adheres to the locality rule, the expert witness must also show familiarity with the standard of care practiced in the defendant's community.

As a general rule, physicians consider the use of expert medical testimony a means of ensuring judgment by their peers—by people knowledgeable about medical science and its inexactness, and with reasonable and realistic expectations of what constitutes good medical practice. Doctors view expert medical testimony as a partial safeguard against emotional judgments based on unfortunate but unforeseeable results.

Res Ipsa Loquitur

There is a special type of professional negligence case in which the plaintiff usually does not need the testimony of an expert medical witness.

These cases are based on the doctrine of *res ipsa loquitur*—"the thing speaks for itself." In some states, this doctrine is known as the "common knowledge doctrine."

In these cases, the plaintiff claims that the circumstantial evidence so clearly indicates the doctor's negligence as the proximate cause of the injury that the judge or jury may presume the defendant liable without expert testimony. When cases are tried under this doctrine, the burden of proof automatically shifts to the defendant, who must prove a lack of negligence or that the negligence did not cause the patient's injury.

During pretrial activities a judge considers the plaintiff's evidence and decides whether the case may be tried on the basis of *res ipsa loquitur*. The judge's decision depends on the existence of three conditions:

1. An injury occurred that could not have occurred unless there was negligence.
2. The defendant had direct control over the apparent cause of the injury.
3. The patient could not have contributed to the injury.

Cases based on the doctrine of *res ipsa loquitur* typically arise from one of the following situations: (1) a foreign object, such as a sponge or instrument, is unintentionally left in the patient's body during surgery; (2) the patient is accidentally burned while anesthetized; (3) some of the patient's healthy tissue is damaged during an operation on another part of his/her body; or (4) the patient suffers an infection caused by the use of unsterilized instruments.

It is certainly to the plaintiff's advantage for a case to be tried under the doctrine of *res ipsa loquitur*. The problem of finding an expert medical witness is usually eliminated, and the costly and time-consuming burden of proof shifts to the defendant.

Damages

When a plaintiff can prove that he/she was injured by the defendant's negligence, the plaintiff is entitled to compensation (known as damages) for the injuries sustained. Indeed, the purpose of most civil lawsuits is the recovery of compensation for injuries caused by a legal wrong—such as negligence, breach of contract, or slander.

The law recognizes three categories of damages:

1. **Nominal damages**—Token compensation awarded when the court wishes to recognize that the plaintiff's legal rights were violated, even though no actual loss was proved by plaintiff. One dollar is the usual token award.
2. **Actual or compensatory damages**—Money awarded for injuries or losses attributable to the violation of the patient's rights. There are two types of actual damages:

   - **General damages**, which represent compensation for the consequences of the wrong—pain and suffering, physical disability, loss of earnings, and loss of the service of a spouse or child. In many cases, the award covers losses incurred to date and anticipated future losses, such as an anticipated increase in earnings the injured party would probably have acquired, as well as future pain and suffering. In professional negligence cases, damages for mental suffering are awarded only when a physical injury occurs.

- **Special damages,** which represent compensation for losses that are caused by the wrong, but are not necessarily a direct consequence of it (e.g., additional medical expenses). The dollar value of certain general damages does not have to be proved. Special damages claimed by the plaintiff must be substantiated and proved.

3. **Punitive damages** (sometimes called exemplary damages)—Compensation awarded beyond actual damages as punishment to the wrongdoer for the reckless or malicious nature of the wrongdoing. Punitive damages are rarely awarded in ordinary negligence suits, unless fraud or some other deliberate misdeed is involved.

The right to recover damages is a question of law. The amount of damages actually awarded is a question of fact and thus is determined by the trier of fact—a jury or, in the case of a bench trial, a judge. The plaintiff must show the existence, nature, and probable duration of any injury for which he/she is claiming damages. The plaintiff has the right to appeal a damage award that is considered inadequate, just as the defendant has the right to appeal a damage award that is considered excessive.

In the late seventies, a jury awarded a man $1,290 for injuries caused by a fluoroscopic spot film device that fell on him while he was undergoing an x-ray examination. The award was earmarked $786 for loss of past earnings and $504 for physical pain and suffering. The plaintiff felt the award was inadequate and appealed. The appellate court upheld the decision, noting that testimony and evidence presented during the trial supported the jury's decision. There was testimony that, at the time of the accident, the patient complained of leg pain, not back pain; that the patient had complained of back injury prior to the accident; that the patient did not see a doctor until eighteen days after the accident; and that he did not complain of back pain until one month after the injury. The court also noted that the patient made considerably more money in the two years after the accident than in the two years before it. *(Partida v Park North General Hospital*, 592 S.W.2d 38, Tex. 1979)

Most health care professionals have professional liability insurance to protect their assets in the event of an adverse decision. Generally, the insurer of a defendant pays any damages awarded the plaintiff to the extent of the insured's policy limits. In addition, most insurers provide experienced defense counsel for their insureds.

Insurance protection is usually limited to unintentional wrongs, such as ordinary negligence. Intentional wrongs, such as permitting laymen to practice medicine without a license and the wrongs discussed in Chapter Eight, are usually not covered.

Wrongful Death Statutes

If a doctor's negligence causes a patient's death, the patient's heirs may recover damages in accordance with state statutes commonly known as wrongful death acts. The purpose of these statutes is to compensate the patient's heirs for losses they incur as a result of the death—e.g., loss of income. Rules governing the litigation of wrongful death claims are similar to the rules governing litigation of ordinary negligence suits.

COMPETENCY CHECK: THREE

10. Why is it necessary for the plaintiff in the typical professional liability suit against a doctor to obtain an expert medical witness?

11. In broad terms, what are the qualifications of an expert medical witness?

12. In a professional negligence suit tried on the doctrine of *res ipsa loquitur*, upon whom is placed the burden of proof?

13. **List and briefly explain three categories of damages recognized by the legal system.**

LAW OF AGENCY

In addition to being liable for their own negligence, doctors are almost always liable for the negligence of employees and agents if the negligence occurs during the course and scope of an individual's employment by the doctor.

Several legal terms, often used interchangeably, express this liability. The most common ones are the doctrine of *respondeat superior*, vicarious liability, and the "captain of the ship" doctrine. All of these concepts are based on the law of agency.

The law of agency governs the legal relationship between two people whenever, by mutual consent, one party (the agent) agrees to act on behalf of the other party (the principal) and the agent's work—method and result—is subject to the control of the principal.

The law of agency applies to the relationship existing between most employers and employees. In addition to stipulating what is to be done and how, employers control employees by supervising their work and through hiring, evaluation, motivation, and disciplinary practices.

The doctrine of *respondeat superior* ("let the master answer") is the legal term or rule used most often to express the liability of a principal/employer for the negligence of an agent/employee. Under this doctrine, a doctor is responsible for the negligence of assistants/ agents/employees when the negligence occurs within the course and scope of the assistants'/agents'/employees' duties. The term "course and scope of employment" limits the doctor's liability to those acts or omissions performed by the employees within the normal course of employment and to the extent of the responsibility (scope of employment) delegated to them.

The liability of the doctor for the negligence of an employee does not immunize that employee from liability.

The law holds everyone liable for his/her own negligence. An injured party may sue the employee as well as the employer. In some instances, an employer or the

employer's insurer may sue an employee to recover
employee-caused damages that the employer had to pay.

Doctors and Their Employees

The employer/employee relationship existing between doctors and their office personnel is certainly an agency relationship. Doctors in private practice have repeatedly been
found liable under the doctrine of *respondeat superior* for
an employee's negligence that occurs during the course and
in the scope of the individual's employment.

> A patient suffered wristdrop because an injection was improp-
> erly administered by a physician's employee. The physician
> was held liable for the employee's negligence. (*Bauer v Otis*,
> 284 P.2d 133, Cal. 1955)

> A physician prescribed a series of injections for his patient.
> According to the patient, the physician said that his office
> assistant would administer the injection if the physician was
> ever unavailable. The patient arrived for an injection one day
> while the physician was on vacation, and the assistant gave the
> injection. A few hours later the patient's arm began to swell,
> and she experienced pain and a high fever. A week later the
> swelling burst, revealing a needle that had broken off during
> the injection. The patient sued the physician for negligence. In
> his defense the physician acknowledged the assistant's negli-
> gence but denied she had the authority to give injections. The
> court held otherwise. It said that the physician implied that the
> patient could rely on the assistant's skill in giving the injection
> because: (1) the physician left the medications and office under
> the control of the assistant; (2) the patient's medication, time,
> and method of delivery were all predetermined by the physi-
> cian; and (3) the physician did not provide a substitute physi-
> cian in his absence. (*Mullins v Du Vall*, 104 S.E.513, Ga. 1920)

To reduce the likelihood of rendering an employer
liable for negligence under the doctrine of *respondeat superior*, as well as to protect his/her own reputation, assets, and
career, an allied health professional should:

 • Clearly understand his/her job responsibilities.
Specific duties should be itemized in a written job

description, which should be updated periodically and kept in the personnel file.

- Never try to perform any procedure for which he/she is not properly trained. If asked to do so by the doctor, the employee should tell the doctor of the inability to perform the procedure.
- Diligently and carefully perform his/her duties. If a mistake is made, tell the employer immediately.

Hospital Employees

Hospital staff nurses, interns, residents, dietitians, aides, assistants, technicians, orderlies, janitors, etc., are normally hired, fired, and paid by hospitals. An agency relationship exists between the hospital as employer and its employees. The hospital is, therefore, usually liable for the negligence of an employee that occurs within the course and scope of the employee's duties.

Doctors in private practice who have staff privileges at local hospitals give hospital employees instructions concerning the care of patients. These doctors have a right to expect that their instructions will be properly carried out, provided the assignment is within the course and scope of each employee's duties. Failure by a hospital employee to carry out routine instructions can render the hospital—not the doctor who gave the instructions—liable for damages.

> A physician left orders that if a certain patient complained of being cold, a hospital nurse should give the patient a heating pad. The patient was burned when the pad was allowed to overheat. In the ensuing lawsuit, the court ruled that the physician had a right to expect the hospital nursing staff to properly perform such simple procedures and, therefore, the physician was not liable. (*Burke v Pearson*, 191 S.E.2d 721, S.C. 1972)

Borrowed Servant Doctrine

When, however, a hospital employee is temporarily "borrowed" by a doctor to perform certain duties under the doctor-borrower's direct supervision and personal control, the doctor is often liable for any negligence by the employee during that period of time. This legal theory is known as the *borrowed servant doctrine*. The situation most commonly covered by this doctrine occurs in operating rooms where surgeons use hospital employees to assist with surgical procedures. Many courts have ruled that, from the time an incision is made to the time the patient is "closed," the surgeon-in-charge is responsible for all that occurs. In some instances, this strict liability has been extended to cover the patient's care in the recovery room.

Doctors/Private Duty Nurses

Private duty nurses are usually considered employees or agents of the patients hiring and paying them. Therefore, a doctor would not be responsible for the negligence of a private duty nurse under the doctrine of *respondeat superior*. If, however, a doctor observed a private duty nurse doing something negligently and failed to stop him/her, the doctor might be found independently negligent.

Doctors/Pharmacists

The doctrine of *respondeat superior* does not apply to the relationship between doctor and pharmacist because an agency relationship does not exist. A doctor would not be liable for the negligence of a pharmacist who makes an error in compounding a prescription, but a doctor would certainly be liable for negligence in writing an incorrect prescription. A pharmacist could be found negligent for filling a prescription that he/she knows—or should know— could injure the patient.

COMPETENCY CHECK: FOUR

14. Briefly define the doctrine of *respondeat superior*.

15. Under what circumstances is a doctor liable for the negligence of an employee?

16. Under what circumstances is a doctor liable for the negligence of a hospital employee?

17. **What two elements must exist before the law of agency applies to a relationship?**

SUMMARY

Failure to act with reasonable care constitutes the tort of negligence—a civil wrong for which the wrongdoer is liable for damages.

A health care professional provides his/her patient with reasonable care when he/she treats the patient with the same degree of knowledge, skill, and care that peers would provide under the same or similar circumstances. This principle, however, is easier to state than to apply.

The vast majority of lawsuits against health care professionals are based on allegations of professional negligence —that the health care provider did not provide reasonable care and that this negligence was the proximate cause of damage or injury to the patient.

The plaintiff in such cases must usually depend on expert medical witnesses to support the allegations. However, there is a special type of professional negligence case in which the plaintiff usually does not need the testimony of an expert witness. These cases are based on the doctrine of *res ipsa loquitur* ("the thing speaks for itself"), also known as the common knowledge doctrine. These suits usually arise from incidents such as a sponge left in a patient's body during surgery or an infection caused by the use of unsterilized instruments.

When the plaintiff proves the allegations of negligence, he/she may receive: (1) nominal damages; (2) actual or compensatory damages; and (3) punitive damages.

In addition to being liable for his/her own negligence, a doctor may be responsible for the negligence of others. Terms often used to express this liability are the doctrine of *respondeat superior*, vicarious liability, and "captain of the ship" doctrine. These terms and concepts are based on the law of agency. The law of agency governs whenever by mutual consent one party (the agent) agrees to act on behalf of the other (the principal), and the agent's work is subject to the control of the principal.

An agency relationship exists between the health care professional and his/her employees. Although the employer may be liable for an employee's negligence, the employee may *also* be held liable and should strive to protect his/her own reputation, career, and assets.

When you have finished reading this chapter, complete the corresponding chapter in your workbook and then go on to Chapter Seven.

REFERENCES

1. Schneider v Little Co., 151 N.W. 587, 588 (Mich. 1915).
2. Herbert AP. *Misleading Cases in the Common Law*. 4th ed. New York, NY: GP Putnam & Sons; 1930:16.
3. Holder AR. *Medical Malpractice Law* 2nd ed. New York, NY: John Wiley and Sons; 1978:59.

7

Defenses to Professional Liability Suits

Defending medical malpractice suits is not easy. It is time-consuming, expensive, often demoralizing for the defendants, and sometimes damaging to their reputations. On the other hand, negligence is no easier to prove than it is to defend.

This chapter focuses on defenses against professional liability suits. It stresses the importance of the patient records in such suits and discusses the denial defense, affirmative defenses, and technical legal defenses.

OBJECTIVES

After studying this chapter, you will be able to:

1. Name and give examples of at least three uses of medical records in professional liability suits.
2. Contrast a denial defense to an affirmative defense.
3. State the purpose of the statute of limitations and some common state policies for determining the beginning of the statutory period.
4. Define and give examples of the following terms: contributory negligence, *res judicata*, and toll.

MEDICAL RECORDS

Medical records, which are key factors in most professional liability suits, have a number of uses.

Well-kept records can help refresh a defendant's memory about a case that may have occurred one, two, three, or even more years earlier. Without such records, a health care professional could be found liable simply because he/she could not recall the patient or the situation. Fairly or not, juries tend to equate loss of recollection and/or loss of records with intentional concealment of wrongdoing.

Well-kept records reflecting adequate care and attention to the patient's problems always support and strengthen a defendant's defense. They may even serve to have a case dismissed before it reaches the trial stage. While patient records are not in themselves proof of reasonable care, well-kept records may help substantiate such care. On the other hand, they may also show a deviation from the standard, thereby documenting the patient's claim. Poorly-kept records, however, always enhance the plaintiff's claim and may work against a defendant, even when the negligence was in record keeping and not in treatment.

> After a difficult labor and delivery, a woman bled so heavily that transfusions were required and eventually a hysterectomy was performed. The patient developed hepatitis from the transfusions. The patient sued the physician for negligence and claimed that if he had attended her during labor, the complications could have been prevented. The physician claimed he was there. However, the hospital chart did not indicate his presence or his monitoring. The judge told the jury it could conclude that monitoring did not occur. (*Stack v Wapner*, 368 A.2d 292, Pa. 1976)

Records are also of critical importance in informed consent cases. The inclusion in the patient's record of a well-detailed and properly executed form would document the defendant's position that the patient knew of the treatment risks and had consented to them prior to treatment.

When a patient record needs to be corrected, a fine, single line should be drawn through the incorrect data, and a marginal note should be made that indicates who made the change, when, and why. The original entry should never be obliterated or removed. The correct information should be added in chronological order.

Changes in medical records after the filing of a professional negligence suit have been construed, by some courts, as attempts to cover up mistakes and avoid liability. Some courts have even ruled that an alteration of records creates a presumption of negligence.

Altering a subpoenaed record, or one that is likely to be subpoenaed, in a deliberate attempt to change the outcome of a lawsuit is a criminal offense.

DENIAL DEFENSE

The defense used most frequently by health professionals is "denial defense." The doctor denies negligence and therefore denies liability for the patient's alleged injury. Since the burden of proof is normally on the plaintiff, the defendant does not have to prove a lack of negligence. He/she may even elect to have the case decided solely on the merits of the plaintiff's evidence.

Normally, however, the defendant will rebut the plaintiff's evidence by testifying and/or presenting the testimony of expert medical witnesses. In doing so, the defendant will attempt to prove that the standard of care was met or exceeded.

AFFIRMATIVE DEFENSES

Instead of simply denying negligence, a defendant may present one of several affirmative defenses. In an affirmative defense, the health care professional presents evidence to show that the patient's condition is due to some cause other than negligence.

Contributory Negligence

"Contributory negligence is conduct on the part of the plaintiff which falls below the standard to which he should conform for his own protection, and which is a legally contributing cause co-operating with the negligence of the defendant in bringing about the plaintiff's harm."[1]

Essentially, the defense claims the injury is at least partly the plaintiff's fault. The classic example used to illustrate this theory is the motorist who runs a red light and hits a speeding motorist. The driver of the first car would claim that the other driver was contributorily negligent.

A doctor might plead contributory negligence as a defense in two types of situations. In one type, the doctor admits negligence, but claims that the patient aggravated the injury through the patient's own negligence. The doctor claims the patient did something a reasonable patient would not have done, or failed to do something a reasonable patient would have done.

In the second type of situation, the defendant-doctor denies any negligence whatsoever and attempts to show that the patient's condition is totally the result of the patient's own actions. (In this situation the term "contributory negligence" is actually a misnomer.)

> A patient was hospitalized after a severe beating. He left the hospital against his physician's advice and, despite instructions to eat only baby food, ate normally and drank alcohol. He died of peritonitis within a day. His widow sued the physician for negligence. The jury found the deceased solely responsible for his own death because of his deliberate failure to follow the physician's directions. No damages were awarded. (*Musachia v Rosman*, 190 So.2d 47, Fla. 1966)

> A physician set a fractured arm and instructed the patient not to use it for picking up heavy objects. The patient tried to pick up a heavy sack, and the arm did not heal. The court ruled that his disregard for the physician's directions precluded a recovery for negligent treatment. (*Shirey v Schlemmer*, 223 N.E.2d 759, Ind. 1967)

Comparative Negligence

In some states, proof of contributory negligence prevents the patient from recovering any damages. An increasing number of states, however, follow the *doctrine of comparative negligence* in professional liability suits and apportion the damages according to the percentage of negligence by each party. If, for example, a court finds that 20 percent of the patient's condition is due to his/her own negligence, the damage award will be reduced by that percentage.

> After a cataract operation, a patient developed an eye infection. She did not keep her appointments with the ophthalmologist

and her eye was permanently damaged. She sued for negligent treatment and was advised by the court that her failure to keep the appointments would not defeat her suit, but would lessen the damage award. (*Heller v Medine*, 377 N.Y.S. 100, 1975)

Ability to Comprehend

In trying professional liability cases in which the defense claims contributory negligence, the court considers the patient's ability to grasp and follow the doctor's instructions. Unconscious patients clearly cannot contribute to their own injuries; young children, senile patients, and mentally ill people would probably not be held liable for their actions. In times of sickness and great pain, even mentally competent adults cannot be expected to exercise the same degree of care and judgment that they would exercise when well.

COMPETENCY CHECK: ONE

1. What information should be noted when a medical record needs correcting?

2. Define contributory negligence.

3. How might a patient's failure to follow a doctor's reasonable instructions be construed?

4. How is the doctrine of comparative negligence applied in professional liability cases?

TECHNICAL DEFENSES

In addition to defenses based on factual matters, a number of technical legal points may prevent a doctor from being found liable for a patient's condition. These legal points are always decided by a judge as a point of law. (Juries—and judges in bench trials—decide questions of fact; judges decide all questions of law.)

Statute of Limitations

The statute of limitations is the time limit set on enforcement of a right through litigation. The time limit varies according to the type of case. The following paragraphs discuss the statute of limitations governing professional negligence suits and breach of contract suits.

Trying a professional liability case fifteen or twenty years after the occurrence of an alleged injury is extremely difficult. Aside from the daunting task of reconstructing what actually transpired, establishing the standard of care of fifteen or twenty years ago is a formidable job.

Every state has, therefore, enacted a law limiting the amount of time an injured party has to file a personal injury lawsuit. A court does not permit a patient to sue a health care provider for professional negligence after this statutory period has expired.

Among the states, statutes of limitations vary greatly—both in length and in ways of determining when the statutory period begins. The more common ways are:

- Occurrence or time of negligence rule. Historically, most states and courts have held that the statutory period begins the day the alleged negligence occurred. If the patient did not discover the negligence within the stipulated time period, he/she had no recourse against a doctor for negligence even if negligence is discovered later. Many states still follow this rule.
- Last treatment rule. A few states have established the beginning date of the statutory period as the last day of the course of treatment. The rationale is that as long as the doctor is treating the patient, the negligence continues.
- Discovery rule. In a substantial number of states, the statutory period begins on the date of "discovery," which is defined as the day a reasonable person discovers—or would have known of—the negligence. The way a patient usually discovers negligence is by consulting another doctor and learning the nature of his/her problem. In such cases, the discovery date is the date the second doctor identifies the problem.

- Combination policy. In an effort to strike a balance, some states have adopted a rather complex way of setting the beginning of the statutory period. This way combines important features of the occurrence rule and the discovery rule. The states adopting a combination policy have:

  o Established a maximum time period within which all medical negligence actions must be filed. This period is often three or four years after occurrence of the alleged negligence.
  o Set a shorter time limit, usually two years, for filing complaints when the patient knew or should have known that negligence occurred immediately or soon after the alleged event.
  o Set an additional time period, usually a year or so, for filing complaints based on injuries discovered some time after occurrence. The court permits a suit in such cases provided the maximum time period has not expired and the patient-plaintiff can establish that a reasonable person would not have discovered the problem any earlier.

Interruption

Almost all states recognize conditions that toll (a legal term for interrupt) or extend the statute of limitations. One is fraudulent concealment by the doctor of the true nature of the patient's condition. Another is the inability of the patient to pursue his/her case because he/she has been declared incompetent, imprisoned, or otherwise confined. A third condition extending the statute is the demonstration that a foreign object was left in the body during surgery, even if the surgery occurred many years earlier. The theory is that a patient would normally find it difficult to detect a foreign object, and consequently should not be penalized by an inflexible application of the statute of limitations.

Minors

In addition to the differences noted above, the statutes of limitations vary greatly with regard to suits by, or on behalf of, minors. Traditionally, minors could bring suit within the statutory period after they reach the age of majority. However, even this tradition is breaking down as the trend toward shortening limitation periods continues. In many states the statutory period for filing suit begins on the minor's 18th or 21st birthday, others apply the adult law, and still others have a modified policy.

Breach of Contract Suits

The statutory periods for filing breach of contract suits tend to be longer than those for filing medical negligence suits. Also, the length of the period often depends on whether the contract is oral or written. When the statute distinguishes between the two forms of contracts, the limitation period for written contracts is usually longer.

COMPETENCY CHECK: TWO

5. Briefly explain the purpose of statutes of limitations.

6. In states that follow the discovery rule, when does the statute of limitations on medical professional liability suits begin?

7. List at least two conditions that toll the statute of limitations in most states.

Res Judicata

Another legal defense is based on the doctrine of *res judicata* ("the thing has been decided"). This rule asserts that once a claim has been legally resolved on the basis of facts, it cannot be retried between the same parties. The theory is best explained in the following examples:

- A patient sues a doctor for professional negligence and loses. The patient cannot sue for breach of contract on the sole basis of evidence presented in the professional negligence suit.

- A doctor sues a patient for an unpaid bill. The patient defends nonpayment on the grounds that the doctor's care was negligent. The court decides in favor of the doctor. The patient cannot then turn around and sue the doctor for professional negligence. If, however, the patient did not claim negligence as a defense, or if the patient did not respond to the suit, the patient may, in most states, sue for professional negligence.

Most attorneys and consultants advise doctors to use extreme caution in suing patients for unpaid bills, especially if the patient's lack of payment may be due to his/her dissatisfaction with the quality of care and if the possibility of negligence exists. Repeated and persistent pleas for payment often irritate a patient to the point of suing; if left alone, the patient probably would have let the matter pass.

SUMMARY

All health care professionals are potential defendants in professional liability suits.

Basic defenses against such suits include the denial defense, affirmative defenses, and technical defenses.

The denial defense is simply that—a denial of the alleged negligence and therefore a denial of liability.

In an affirmative defense, the health care professional presents factual evidence to show that the patient's condition is due to a cause other than negligence on the part of the professional. An example of an affirmative defense is contributory negligence on the part of the plaintiff.

There are also a number of technical defenses that may prevent a health care professional from being found liable for a patient's injury. A common technical defense is the expiration of the statute of limitations.

A key factor in any professional liability suit is the quality of the patient's medical record. A carelessly kept record always reflects adversely on the person having to defend it.

When you have finished this chapter, complete the corresponding chapter in your workbook and then proceed to Chapter Eight.

REFERENCES

1. Restatement, Second, Torts § 463.

8

Intentional Torts and Criminal Offenses

Approximately 85 percent of all suits against physicians are based on the tort of negligence. Ordinary negligence is an unintentional tort, a mistake made in good faith. Another ten percent of all suits allege assault and battery on the basis that the patient's valid consent to treatment was not obtained. The usual allegation is lack of informed consent. Assault and battery suits based on lack of informed consent are unintentional torts and are tried in much the same way as ordinary negligence actions. These cases have been covered thoroughly in earlier chapters. This chapter focuses on intentional torts and criminal offenses.

All the legal offenses discussed in this chapter have one element in common: they are considered deliberate or intentional misdeeds that violate the rights of an individual and/or the state. While some of these wrongs may be committed unintentionally, the laws of the United States uphold the principle that citizens have the legal duty to know their responsibilities toward others.

OBJECTIVES

After studying this chapter, you will be able to:

1. List and give examples of four intentional torts.
2. Explain the differences between the following terms: defamation of character, libel, and slander.
3. Discuss the tort of fraud and its relationship to the fiduciary nature of the physician–patient relationship.
4. List four characteristics distinguishing crimes from torts.

INTENTIONAL TORTS

Intentional torts are those misdeeds considered to be deliberate wrongs or violations of an individual's legal rights. Ordinarily, actions considered to be deliberate torts do not involve medical treatment, but arise from the physical and private nature of the relationships between health care providers and patients. Since lawsuits alleging deliberate wrongs normally have nothing to do with the quality of medical care administered, neither plaintiffs nor defendants use expert medical testimony to justify their positions. Damages caused by intentional torts usually are not covered by professional liability insurance policies because the damages could easily have been avoided if the physician (or other health care professional) had simply respected the patient's rights.

Assault and Battery

Everyone has the legal right to be free of contact from another. To threaten and impose contact on another without that person's consent is assault and battery, an offense subject to legal redress. Assault is the threat to, or attempt to, touch another. Battery is the unlawful touching itself. (Surgery without the patient's permission is technically a "battery.") The charge of assault and battery may be an unintentional tort, an intentional tort, and/or a criminal offense.

Recall from Chapters Three and Five that no matter how ill a patient is or how effective or necessary the proposed treatment, the patient has the right to refuse it. Forcing a patient to accept treatment can be justified legally only when the patient's refusal will harm someone else.

> While involuntarily confined to a mental hospital for 60 days, a woman was given tranquilizers despite her repeated objections for religious reasons. She was not found mentally ill or incompetent during her confinement, and upon her release she sued the hospital and physician involved for assault and battery. The court found in her favor and said that medication may be given over religious objections only when a patient is harmful to himself or others. (*Winters v Miller*, 517, F.2d 1337, CCA 2, 1975)

On rare occasions, a physician has used physical force on a patient in a way that constituted a deliberate violation of the patient's rights. The law considers this type of force an intentional tort which often results in high damage awards.

> A physician wanted to remove sutures from a small child's toes. The child's mother was told to hold the child in a prone position on the examining table. When the child resisted, the physician spanked her so severely that visible bruises remained for three weeks. The child's mother sued the physician for assault and battery, and the jury found in her favor, a verdict which was upheld in appellate court. (*Burton v Leftwich*, 123 So.2d 766, La. 1960)

> A medical student was attempting to treat a 23-month-old child's lacerated tongue when the child bit the student's finger. The child would not release her hold on the finger, despite numerous pleas and inducements, and finally the student slapped her cheek to force her mouth open. The technique worked, but the parents sued for assault and battery. The jury did not award any damages because the slapping was not done in malice and it did not injure the child, and the appellate court affirmed. (*Mattocks v Bell*, 194 A.2d 307, D.C. 1963)

In a suit based on assault and battery as a deliberate tort, the plaintiff must prove the impermissible touching took place. Since the plaintiff's charge has nothing to do with medical treatment or with the standard of care, expert medical testimony is not required.

The deliberate physical or sexual attack on a patient may render the physician liable not only for damages, but also for criminal sanctions.

COMPETENCY CHECK: ONE

1. A physician tells an employee to give a certain injection to a frail but mentally competent adult patient. When the employee approaches the patient to inject the medication, the patient tells the employee she doesn't want it. If the employee gives the injection over the patient's objections, what could the employee be sued for?

2. Define the following terms: assault, battery.

Defamation of Character

Defamation of character is the tort of damaging a person's character, name, or reputation. If the defamatory statements are written and/or broadcast, such statements constitute the tort of libel. If defamatory statements are oral, they constitute the tort of slander. In order to win a lawsuit for defamation, the plaintiff must prove the following three points:

1. The disclosure by the defendant was false and malicious.
2. The disclosure was made by the defendant to a third party.
3. The plaintiff suffered some type of loss as a result of the defendant's action.

Physicians must be especially careful to avoid making health-related statements which could be construed as having immoral connotations. For example, incorrectly reporting that an unmarried woman is pregnant might be considered defamatory, whereas a similar statement about a married woman might not be. Saying that someone had a broken arm would, in most cases, not be considered defamatory, but disclosing a sexually transmitted disease or mental illness might be.

A physician was treating a teenage girl for a foot infection. He recommended that she be confined to bed and that the services of a home tutor be sought from the school district. The medical report to the school describing the need for the home tutor incorrectly indicated the girl was pregnant. Despite repeated requests from the girl's parents to correct this error, the physician did not cooperate, except to say he would correct it on the school's copy of the report if the parents would bring it to him. Since the school would not release its copy to the parents and since the physician would not request it himself, the error was not rectified. The girl's father sued the physician for libel and was awarded $7,000 in damages. The court said that while the original mistake was probably a good faith mistake, the physician's refusal to correct it merited the suit. (*Vigil v Rice*, 397 P.2d 719, N.M. 1964)

A registered nurse attended a party catered by one of her employer's patients. This patient did not have, and had never had, syphilis, but she did have a condition that repeatedly produced a false positive Wasserman. The physician was aware of this condition. The nurse, however, told the party's hostess that the caterer had syphilis, a communication that ruined the caterer's business. The court permitted the caterer's suit for slander against the nurse. (*Schessler v Keck*, 271 P.2d 588, Cal. 1954)

False Imprisonment

The tort of false imprisonment is the unlawful detention or restraint of someone. Within the scope of health care delivery, most charges of false imprisonment arise from patients being involuntarily committed to mental institutions or to hospital psychiatric wards. (The term "false commitment" is used by some states and scholars. While this term more aptly describes the nature of the offense, most states and reference works still refer to the offense as "false imprisonment.")

If the commitment is the result of a good faith error in diagnosis, the physician may be liable for negligence. If, however, the commitment is a deliberate act based on malice or disregard for statutory commitment procedures, the physician may be liable for the tort of false imprisonment. This is a much more serious matter, one that often results in large damage judgments and occasionally results in criminal prosecution.

To prove a charge of false imprisonment, the plaintiff must show he/she was mentally competent at the time of detention and that the commitment was the result of malice, lack of good faith, or failure to comply with statutory regulations, including a proper examination.

After his wife announced her plans to divorce him, a man had a psychiatrist come to their home "to examine his wife." She later testified that she was not aware of being examined and never agreed to it. Shortly thereafter, the psychiatrist and another physician, who had never seen the woman, signed a statement that she was mentally ill. She was forcibly taken to a psychiatric hospital, owned by the psychiatrist, and involuntarily confined for several weeks. Among other restrictions, she was not allowed to use a telephone and specifically denied permission to call an attorney or call her brother. An injection was administered over her objections and physical resistance. Eventually she found an unlocked telephone and called her brother who arranged for immediate release. She sued the psychiatrist for false imprisonment and was awarded $40,000. The court said that the manner of her commitment was also grounds for false arrest and that the administering of an injection over her objections was assault and battery. (*Stowers v Wolodzko*, 191 N.W.2d 355, Mich. 1971)

Disputes arose between two physicians who were the principal stockholders in a private hospital. The medical staff withdrew staff privileges from one of the physicians, but he soon obtained a court order permitting him access to his patients. That same day, the other physician filed a lunacy complaint against the ousted physician, which caused him to be arrested, examined and detained for several hours. The ousted physician's wife (he was now dead) sued the other for false imprisonment, and the court found in her favor. No evidence was presented during the trial to indicate the ousted physician was ever mentally ill, but there was considerable evidence to indicate spite and malice on the part of the physician filing the lunacy complaint. (*Pendleton v Burkhalter*, 432 S.W.2d 724, Tex. 1968)

All states have enacted statutes governing the involuntary commitment of patients to mental hospitals or facilities. These statutes are briefly discussed in Chapter Nine. Not complying with statutes governing commitment practices is considered direct evidence of lack of good faith and a deliberate violation of a patient's rights. These serious charges always exceed the definition of ordinary negligence and subject the offending physician to a charge of false imprisonment.

Not all suits for false imprisonment stem from situations concerning someone's mental competence. Detaining patients for not paying their bills is a civil wrong that has resulted in successful false imprisonment actions. There are legal ways to collect an unpaid bill. However, detaining a person without a warrant or restricting his/her freedom to move about is not one of them. The involuntary detention of a mentally competent patient, for almost any reason, could be considered false imprisonment.

Fraud in the Fiduciary Relationship

A fraudulent or deceitful act is one performed to intentionally and deliberately misrepresent or conceal the true nature of a situation. (The terms "fraud" and "deceit" are synonymous in most legal applications. One state will use fraud while another may use deceit to describe the same misdeed.) The fiduciary nature of the physician–patient relationship legally obligates physicians to disclose fully and voluntarily to patients all facts that might have a bearing on their conditions. This principle was explained with regard to informed consent, but it also applies to information the physician acquires during and after treatment.

A physician could be charged with fraud or deceit for:

- Deliberately minimizing the true nature of a patient's injuries or intentionally raising false expectations for a complete recovery.
- Assuring a patient that a procedure involves no serious risks when the physician knows otherwise.
- Advising a patient to have unnecessary or worthless surgery. When it has been shown that the advice was motivated by the physician's desire to enhance his/her economic position, damage awards have been large.
- Misrepresenting the nature of a procedure or any relevant facts either before or after treatment.
- Not voluntarily disclosing a mistake to a patient.
- Intentionally misrepresenting or concealing his/her own or a colleague's negligence. In many situations, silence constitutes fraud.

A gynecologist supposedly performed a tubal ligation on a patient, but learned the next day that no tissue from the patient's tubes appeared in the pathology sample. The gynecologist neither informed the patient of the situation nor warned her that she could become pregnant. Three years later she delivered a baby and shortly thereafter sued the physician for negligence. He defended on the basis of an expired statute of limitations, but the court upheld the woman's right to sue and made the following points: (1)

the fiduciary nature of the physician–patient relationship obligated the physician to disclose the facts; (2) silence constituted fraudulent concealment; and (3) the discovery rule would be used to determine the beginning date of the statutory period, and therefore the statutory period had not expired. (*Hardin v Farris*, 530 P.2d 407, N.M. 1974)

A woman was severely burned by radiation therapy. Her husband asked the patient's family physician, who had recommended the radiologist and was responsible for her follow-up care, if the burns were caused by negligence. The family physician said definitely not and that the woman's hypersensitivity was the cause. During one of fifteen hospital stays required for corrective surgery, the woman overheard a physician say to some students that her burns were "the sort of thing that happened when the radiologist puts a patient on the table and goes out to have a cup of coffee." Shortly thereafter the woman changed physicians and sued the radiologist for negligence and all physicians involved for fraud and conspiracy in misrepresenting the cause of her injuries. Although the trial judge dismissed her suit, the appellate court said the trial judge erred and that the woman had a right to trial by jury. The court said, "A physician has the duty to disclose to his patients the facts of a case, and silence is sufficient to constitute fraud." (*Lopez v Sawyer*, 300 A.2d 563, N.J. 1973)

Recall from Chapter Two that a health care professional who commits a fraudulent act may have his/her license revoked, in addition to being sued.

Abortion Fraud

Abortion fraud cases involve women who were tested, told they were pregnant, and given an "abortion"—even though they were not pregnant.

Insurance Fraud

The Federal False Claims Amendments Act of 1986 offers financial incentives to informants in order to uncover Medicaid and Medicare fraud. Many insurance companies offer rewards, install hotlines, hire investigators, and prosecute physicians for a wide spectrum of fraudulent activities.

- Billing for services that were not rendered; billing for procedures that were performed but not needed.
- Writing fraudulent diagnoses or changing dates so that patients will be able to collect for noncompensable care.
- Billing for services provided by another health care provider that are not collectible unless performed by the doctor.
- Billing for a full fee when deductible and copayments are being waived. Insurance companies state that the amount should be the original fee minus any waived deductible and/or copayments.
- Soliciting or accepting kickbacks, bribes, or rebates for services rendered and billed to Medicare or Medicaid.
- Using inappropriate codes for billing (e.g., billing a routine limited visit using an intermediate or comprehensive code.)

Even though employees or other health care providers do not benefit from the fraudulent activities, they can be found guilty of conspiring to commit fraud if circumstances warrant. Licensed health care professionals who are convicted of fraud can lose their licenses to practice.

COMPETENCY CHECK: TWO

3. A patient is involuntarily committed to a mental hospital. Upon his release he decides to sue the physician for false imprisonment. To have a legitimate case, what would he have to show?

4. A surgeon inadvertently left a sponge in a patient during exploratory surgery, a fact that he realized shortly after the operation was completed. If he voluntarily admits his mistake to the patient within a reasonable amount of time, what may he be liable for? If he does not disclose the error, what may he be liable for?

Invasion of Privacy

Closely related to the patient's right to confidentiality is the patient's right to privacy. This right is recognized by statute or common law in almost every state. It entitles an individual to be free of harassment, unwanted publicity, commercial exploitation, and intrusion into his/her personal life. With regard to medical treatment, this means that the patient's explicit written consent must be obtained before:

- Publicity is given the patient's condition. The word "publicity" includes publication of the patient's case in scientific journals, and in public or mass media.

   Plastic surgery was performed on a patient's nose. An article entitled "The Saddlenose" and containing before and after photographs was published in a medical journal without the patient's knowledge or consent. The patient sued the surgeons on the grounds of invasion of privacy for financial gain. The court allowed recovery and said that even a scientific article "may be nothing more than someone's advertisement in disguise." (*Griffin v Medical Society of the State of New York*, 11 N.Y.S. 2d 109, 1939)

   Patients also have the right to limit publicity given their cases, and many choose to restrict publication to scientific purposes. The following case illustrates what can happen when the patient's authorization is exceeded.

   A patient whose baby was to be delivered by Caesarean section agreed to the filming of the birth for showing at a medical meeting. The film footage was later incorporated into a longer film on birth and was shown commercially. The patient was permitted to sue for invasion of privacy. (*Feeney v Young*, 181 N.Y.S. 481, 1920)

- Photographs of a patient are taken (even if publication is not intended) or published.

   A patient with cancer of the larynx permitted his surgeon to take many photographs of him during the course of treatment. The patient understood that the photographs were for the surgeon's private records and not for publication. The patient was hospitalized during the terminal stage of his illness. A few hours before he died, the surgeon came to take more pictures and did so despite the protest of the patient's wife and an indication by the patient that he did not want his picture taken. The patient's widow was allowed to sue the surgeon for assault (he had moved the patient's head for a better camera angle) and invasion of privacy. (*Estate of Berthiaume v Pratt*, 365 A.2d 792, Me. 1976)

The editors and publishers of most biomedical journals require that properly executed consent forms accompany all photographs of identifiable patients submitted for publication. While state laws vary in their requirements, many publishers also insist upon having the consent of both parents (regardless of their marital status) or the child's legal guardian before publishing photographs of minors.

The practice of retouching a photograph in order to block out a patient's eyes or other distinguishing body features is a practice no longer followed by most publishers, unless a patient stipulates it as a condition for consent. This procedure never eliminates the need to obtain the patient's proper consent.

- Observers are permitted during the doctor's examination or treatment.

Accompanied by a friend, a doctor went to a patient's home to deliver her baby. The friend was present during the delivery. The court found that the doctor violated the woman's right to privacy by permitting the presence of his friend. (*De May v Roberts*, 9 N.W. 146, Mich. 1981)

For examples of appropriate consent forms, we turn again to *Medicolegal Forms with Legal Analysis*. One example is shown here in Figure 8-A. Note the specificity and extensiveness of the information required by the form.

Figure 8-A. Sample Authorization to Admit Observers

Patient _____ Place _____ Date _____

I authorize Dr. _____ and the _____ Hospital
to permit the presence of such observers as they may deem fit
to admit in addition to physicians and hospital personnel, while I
am undergoing (operative surgery) (childbirth), examination, and
treatment.

Witness _____ Signed _____

Source: Medicolegal Forms with Legal Analysis, *1973 ed, published by the American Medical Association. Reprinted with permission.*

A patient's right to privacy has also been interpreted to cover the right to be free of harassment:

> A patient died during treatment by a specialist. Shortly there-after, her family received a notice from the office of her family doctor that it was time for her regular checkup. The patient's widower sent a letter to the family doctor informing him that his wife had died and that the notice regarding the checkup was disturbing to him and his children. A short time later the wid-ower filed a wrongful death suit against the family doctor, pre-sumably for not diagnosing his wife's condition promptly. After that the family received two more checkup reminders from the family doctor's office; they subsequently filed suit for invasion of privacy and harassment. The court said that while sending the first notice was probably due to negligence, sending the lat-ter two constituted legitimate grounds for invasion of the family's privacy. (*McCormick v Haley*, 307 N.E.2d 34, Ohio 1973)

Patients also have the right to receive fair and respectful treatment. Eventually all physicians have to deal with indi-viduals from different races, ethnic groups, religions, socioeconomic levels, and age groups. Quality care must be provided for individuals who are homeless, HIV positive or AIDS-inflicted, or practicing alternative lifestyles. All patients must be treated with courtesy and respect.

5. **True or false. As long as the physician does not intend to publish pictures of a patient, the physician does not have to obtain the patient's permission to photograph any physical manifestation of the patient's disease.**

6. **True or false. An obstetrician who permits unauthorized and unessential medical personnel to observe his/her patient during childbirth without obtaining the patient's permission may be sued by the patient for invasion of privacy.**

Undue Influence

Undue influence is the improper coercion of another person in a way that destroys that person's freedom to act.

Most cases of undue influence by health care providers stem from allegations that the provider inaptly influenced the patient (usually one that is senile, mentally incompetent, or terminally ill) to do something for the provider's economic gain (e.g., leaving a substantial sum in a will or selling something for considerably less than fair market value).

> A psychoanalyst treated an elderly woman for many years. During treatment she gave the analyst $116,050, and she also left him a large amount of money in her will. Part of the $116,050 was for professional fees, part for a loan which was never repaid, and $30,000 was a gift. The patient's heirs believed the analyst used undue influence and sought, therefore, to recover all money except professional fees. The court ordered a hearing and the burden of proof was on the analyst to show that the transfers were "fair, open, voluntary, and well understood." (*Estate of Reiner,* 383 N.Y.S.2d 504, 1976)

The allegation of undue influence is easier to avoid than to defend because when a transaction is legally challenged, the recipient of the gift has the burden of proving that undue influence was not applied. Health care professionals should seek legal advice whenever:

- an elderly, senile, or mentally incompetent patient indicates his/her intention to will the health care professional something of value;

- a patient whose intelligence or mental competency is doubtful to any degree offers to sell something at a less-than-fair-market price;
- the patient's family objects to a transaction proposed by the health care professional.

Tort of Outrage

Recently, the courts have recognized a new type of civil wrong known as the tort of intentional infliction of emotional distress. Under this theory, health care providers can be held liable for emotional injuries caused by their "outrageous" behavior, regardless of whether a physical injury occurs. (Historically, damages for emotional injuries were awarded only when a physical injury had also occurred.)

This new theory is tied to two trends in the law. The first is the trend toward holding the health care professional responsible for identifying all reasonably foreseeable injuries, both emotional and physical, related to the patient's condition. The other trend is the court's increasing recognition and expansion of liability for emotional injuries.

To prevail in a lawsuit alleging intentional affliction of emotional distress, the plaintiff must prove four points:

1. The wrongdoer's actions were intentional or reckless; the wrongdoer knew or should have known that his/her behavior would cause emotional distress.
2. The wrongdoer's behavior violated generally-accepted standards of decency and morality.
3. The wrongdoer's actions were the proximate cause of the emotional distress.
4. The emotional distress was severe.

An infant, mother, and grandmother were injured in an automobile accident. The infant's injuries were serious. A doctor whose office was close to the accident scene agreed to meet them in his office and provide treatment. However, when they arrived, the physician refused to examine the unconscious infant. He finally consented, but performed a negligent, superficial examination. He provided no treatment and said nothing was wrong with the child, despite contrary evidence. He was rude, inhuman, and made them wait for the child's father outside the office in below-freezing, stormy weather. The child's father took her immediately to a hospital where she was admitted and hospitalized for over a week. The mother sued the physician for emotional distress caused by his refusal to treat the child. (*Rockhill v Pollard,* 485 P.2d 28, Or. 1971)[1]

COMPETENCY CHECK: FOUR

7. A terminally ill patient, who is generally thought to be "well off," arrives for an appointment with the medical assistant's physician-employer. The medical assistant has helped this patient cope with her illness in several ways, and the patient says to the medical assistant, "Don't worry about your future, dear, I've taken care of you in my will." What, if any, legal actions should the medical assistant take?

Duress

Persuading or coercing a patient (or anyone) physically or verbally, by threat or through pressure, to do something he/she does not want to do constitutes the tort of duress. Duress invalidates consent, and a patient whose consent was obtained through duress may also sue for assault and battery.

There have been reports in public media of welfare patients being coerced into accepting sterilization. When these reports are accurate, the patients have legitimate actions for duress against the parties who forced the consents, and for assault and battery against all involved, including the doctors who performed the procedures and the hospitals in which they were performed.

Malicious Betrayal of Professional Secrets

The doctor–patient relationship is a confidential one, and except for disclosures required or authorized by law, doctors must refrain from discussing patients with third parties. The doctor who violates this confidence commits a tort. The action may be called a breach of confidence, breach of contract, or invasion of privacy, depending on the circumstances and the jurisdiction in which the complaint is filed.

In considering a tort action based on breach of confidence, the courts take into consideration whether the breach was a good faith mistake or the malicious betrayal of a professional secret. The former would be considered an unintentional wrong entitling the plaintiff to compensatory damages only, but the latter would be an intentional tort that could very well subject the doctor to punitive damages, license revocation, and criminal prosecution.

CRIMINAL OFFENSES

The vast and extremely complex subject of criminal law is given only brief attention in this book. A basic understanding of this subject is of professional and personal importance to health care professionals.

Criminal offenses are distinguishable from torts in many ways. The basic distinctions are as follows:

- Acts classified as criminal offenses are specifically established and carefully defined by state or federal statute, while offenses classified as torts are defined only generally in statutory law and are usually subject to judicial interpretation.

   A criminal offense is the commission of an act forbidden by law or the omission of an act required by law.

   Agents of an insurance company covertly obtained confidential medical information from a hospital over the telephone. The agents then gave the information to the insurance company. A state district attorney learned of the incident and attempted to charge the insurance company with theft, claiming that the confidential information was a "thing of value." The trial court dismissed the case, a decision upheld by the state supreme court. It said that the state legislature could have made the violation of medical privacy a criminal offense but had not done so. While both courts condemned the conduct of the insurance company and its agents, they ruled their actions were not criminal according to state law. (*People v Home Ins. Co.*, 591 P.2d 1036, Colo. 1979)

- Crimes are considered offenses against the state and/or the public welfare; torts are wrongs against individuals. The state prosecutes criminal offenders, but persons against whom a tortious act has been committed must file suit to obtain legal redress.

- The prosecutor in a criminal case must prove the defendant "guilty beyond a reasonable doubt;" the plaintiff in a civil action must prove his/her case by a "preponderance of evidence."

  The same act may subject a person to both criminal prosecution and a civil suit, yet because of different procedural rules, the person could be acquitted of a criminal charge yet be liable in a civil suit. The reverse is also possible, but less likely.

- Crimes are classified as misdemeanors or felonies. Misdemeanors are less serious offenses resulting in less serious penalties, such as fines. Felonies are considered major crimes, punishable by imprisonment for one or more years. Examples include murder, rape, and burglary.

The following discussion of criminal offenses addresses some of those crimes that occur within the course of health care delivery.

Murder

Defined as the unlawful killing of a human being with intent to kill, murder is the most serious criminal charge. Lawmakers distinguish between first-degree murder and second-degree murder. The former is an unlawful killing that is willful and deliberate. Second-degree murder is an unlawful killing that is willful, but without deliberation, such as what might occur during a violent argument.

Fetal Murder

A 1994 California Supreme Court ruling gave California the toughest fetal murder law in the country.[2] Prosecutors may charge a defendant with murder for causing a pregnant woman to miscarry, even if the fetus is only eight weeks old and unable to survive outside the uterus. This ruling has raised the question of whether someone can be convicted for killing a nonviable fetus that can be *legally* aborted.

Euthanasia

Euthanasia, mercy killing, and assisted suicide have been receiving wide media coverage. Victims of Alzheimer's disease and AIDS have pleaded with friends and family for relief from the ravages of their diseases. At the present time, there are no clear-cut guidelines and no consistency in the way authorities handle cases. Various state legislatures are attempting to pass laws regarding these matters, and courts are wrestling with the constitutional (federal and state), statutory, and common law dimensions of these issues.

Manslaughter

Murder must be distinguished from manslaughter, which is the unlawful killing of a human being with no malice or intent to kill. Most charges of manslaughter against health care personnel arise from conduct so grossly negligent that it results in a patient's death. Consider the following case:

> A nurse was instructed by a surgeon to prepare an anesthetic of 10 percent cocaine solution with adrenaline. After the medication was injected, the patient died. Although the surgeon meant to say procaine rather than cocaine, the nurse did not question his order. By virtue of her education, training and experience she should have known better, and her failure to question constituted gross negligence. She was charged with and convicted of manslaughter.[3]

Although the physician acted negligently in the foregoing case, the nurse was charged criminally because her act was the one that caused the patient's death. Every person is responsible for his/her own actions. Ordinary negligence is never considered a criminal offense, but when the negligence is so willful, careless, or reckless that it suggests a disregard for life or human welfare, it may be treated as criminal negligence.

Sexual Assault and Battery/Rape

The deliberate sexual attack on a patient may result in criminal charges of assault and battery and/or rape. Telling a patient that sexual intercourse is a part of medical or psychiatric treatment may be considered "rape by fraud;" it has never been successfully defended as within the realm of due care. Having sexual intercourse after medicating a patient to an unconscious state may be considered forcible rape.

The most subtle hint of sexual misconduct is so potentially damaging to doctors that they carefully avoid situations from which such a charge might arise. Many do this by having an associate or employee present during certain types of examinations.

Practicing Medicine Without a License

An issue of concern to nonphysician health providers is the distinction between giving first aid and practicing medicine without a license. The latter, no matter how successful, can be prosecuted criminally. The American Red Cross and the American Medical Association have identified actions that do not constitute the practice of medicine (See the American Red Cross first aid handbook.) First aid has been defined as immediate and temporary care given to a victim until the services of a physician or other qualified personnel can be obtained. Many health care facilities have "standing orders" or protocols for emergency room personnel.

COMPETENCY CHECK: FIVE

8. State the difference between murder and manslaughter.

9. List three ways in which crimes and torts differ.

Domestic Violence

Child Abuse
In 1987, Congress passed the Federal Child Abuse Prevention and Treatment Act. In addition, every state has legisla-

tion concerning the crime of child abuse. Child abuse is defined as "mistreatment of a child by a parent or other responsible caretaker that causes injury or harm or puts the child at risk of injury or harm." Neglect is defined as "failure to provide adequate food, clothing, shelter or other basics for a child."

Child abuse laws mandate reporting of suspected cases of child abuse or neglect and list those individuals who are mandated as reporters. For example, physicians, other health care providers, and school personnel are designated reporters. In an ambulatory facility, the physician should be the appropriate person to report, unless another member of the staff has been assigned that task. In a legal brief in the *PMA*, Donald A. Balasa, JD, MBA, executive director and legal counsel for the AAMA, stated that: "Informing a superior of suspected child abuse is often insufficient. For example, a(n) . . . assistant would not fulfill her/his duties under most states if she/he reported suspected abuse to the supervising physician but not to the state."[4]

The report should be made immediately, and certainly before the child/victim is returned to the care of the suspected abuser.

In most states, a physician who in good faith reports a suspicion of child abuse is immune from suit for negligence or defamation of character if the suspicion is not confirmed. On the other hand, a physician who fails to report a suspected case may be held criminally and civilly liable.

Suppose a physician suspects that a child's injuries are the result of abuse, but does not report his/her suspicions to the proper authorities. Suppose further that the child returns to his/her home and suffers another abusive beating. The physician's failure to report may be considered the proximate cause of the child's subsequent injuries because if the report had been made, the home situation would have been investigated before the child was returned.

A one-year-old child was treated in an emergency room for a fractured leg and other injuries. The nature of the injuries suggested abuse, but the treating physician made no report. Shortly thereafter, the child was admitted again for serious and permanent injuries obviously caused by an abusive beating. The child was taken from her parents and a guardian appointed. The guardian attempted to sue the first physician for failure to report the original incident, and the court upheld her cause of action. *(Landeros v Flood,* 131 CA Rptr 69, *Cal. Rptr. Supp.* 1976)

Generally, the parents of a minor enter into the patient–doctor relationship and are entitled to the right of confidentiality. But, in the case of suspected child abuse, it has been held that the child—not the parents—is the patient, and that the duty of confidentiality is owed the child. During investigation of the situation, the confidentiality privilege is held by the investigating agency and release of information must be given by that agency. If the agency refers the complaint to the district attorney, it becomes a criminal case.

In some states, other mandated reporters include day care and preschool personnel as well as all other officers of the court, such as probation officers and social workers. Additionally, any individual may report suspected cases of child abuse to the child protective agencies.

In child abuse cases, physicians must realize that the *child*—not the parents—is their primary responsibility. Their legal obligation is to act in the child/patient's best interests. Methods of reporting also vary from state to state. Familiarize yourself with the child abuse laws in your state.

Abuse of the Elderly and Dependent Adults

Abuse of the elder or dependent adult can include the following: (a) physical abuse, which includes: assault, battery, assault with a deadly weapon or force likely to produce great bodily harm; unreasonable physical constraint or prolonged or continued deprivation of food or water; or sexual assault; (b) neglect; (c) intimidation; (d) cruel punishment; (e) fiduciary abuse (a person with custody improperly obtaining money or property of dependent adult or elder); (f) other treatment resulting in physical harm or pain; and (g) deprivation by a care custodian of goods or services necessary to avoid physical harm or mental suffering.

Elders are individuals 65 years of age or older. Dependent adults are individuals between the ages of 18 and 64 who have physical or mental limitations that restrict their ability to carry out normal activities or protect their rights, and persons who are admitted as inpatients in an acute care hospital or other 24-hour facility, as defined by law.

Spousal Abuse

Most states do not have laws that mandate the reporting of spouse abuse, or other forms of family violence. This may change in the next few years as a result of the growing awareness of the frequency and severity of domestic violence other than child abuse. The death of Nicole Brown Simpson and the subsequent trial of O.J. Simpson has forced domestic violence to the forefront of national awareness. Some legislative reforms are likely to follow.

Embezzlement

Embezzlement is defined as the unlawful taking of the property of another by a party entrusted with the property. Embezzlement is not the same as robbery because there is no taking by the use of force or fear. In the health care office setting, the embezzler is often a longtime trusted employee. It is not uncommon for a person terminated for embezzlement by one medical or dental office to get another job in a health care office and embezzle again.

For a variety of reasons, doctors frequently do not withhold references or press charges. Some physicians do not want to admit that they have been victimized. The criminal trial of the embezzler can be a long process, and it is rarely possible to recover fully from the embezzler.

Legal and health care authorities have urged physicians to develop better internal controls and to press charges if they are victimized. An oncologist writing for *Medical Economics* offered the following insights:

> What have I learned from experience? That *all* billing systems require careful monitoring. While Kay had used my computer as an accomplice, she could just as easily have tinkered with

the ledger I'd used before. Her scam was a simple one: It hinged on making false adjustments and issuing fake receipts. You can't let camaraderie lull you into abandoning your responsibility to oversee your staff. It's tempting to let your guard down when employees feel like family—but that can be a costly mistake.[5]

Statutory Offenses

The federal government and each state have enacted a number of statutes governing the performance of certain medical procedures, such as prescribing narcotics, performing autopsies, and committing patients to mental hospitals. A violation of these statutes may result in criminal prosecution. As these statutes govern what are commonly known as the health care professional's public responsibilities, they will be discussed in greater detail in the next chapter, "Public Duties and Responsibilities."

COMPETENCY CHECK: SIX

10. True or false: Almost every state, as well as the federal government, has passed legislation concerning the crime of child abuse.

11. True or false: Statutes identify health care providers, school personnel, and usually probation officers, social workers, and day care and preschool staff members as required reporters of suspected cases of child abuse or neglect.

12. True or false: A doctor who fails to report a case of suspected child abuse, elder abuse, or dependent adult abuse can be held criminally and civilly liable.

13. True or false: In child abuse cases, physicians must realize that the parents, not the child, are their primary concern.

14. True or false: Health care providers are being urged not only to report all forms of domestic violence, but to help identify potential future abusive situations in order to facilitate intervention and prevention.

15. True or false: Embezzlement in private dental, medical, and veterinary offices has been more widespread than formerly believed.

SUMMARY

The great majority of suits against doctors are based on the tort of negligence—an *unintentional* tort. This chapter, however, looked at the problems of *intentional* torts and criminal offenses.

Intentional torts range from assault and battery to intentional infliction of emotional distress, malicious betrayal of professional secrets, duress, defamation of character, false imprisonment, fraud or deceit, and undue influence.

Assault and battery is a common legal offense. The cause of action is based on every person's right to be free of unwanted contact with another and arises from touching a person without permission. Assault is the threat of touching, or the attempt to touch, another. Battery is the deed itself. Coercing someone to do what he/she does not want to do constitutes the tort of duress. Such duress invalidates consent, which can give rise to a charge of assault and battery.

Malicious betrayal of professional secrets and defamation of character are serious breaches of legal duties. The former, for example, can result in punitive damages, license revocation, and criminal prosecution.

False imprisonment situations relate mainly to the involuntary commitment of a patient to a mental institution or to a hospital's psychiatric ward. False imprisonment is a serious matter that can result in large damage judgments and, on occasion, criminal prosecution.

The fiduciary nature of the doctor-patient relationship legally obligates the doctor to disclose fully and voluntarily all facts that might have a bearing on the patient's condition. To intentionally do otherwise constitutes fraud or deceit.

A new type of civil wrong is now being recognized in many jurisdictions. Under this new theory, health care professionals can be held liable for emotional injuries caused by their "outrageous" behavior, regardless of whether a physical injury occurs. Historically, damages for emotional injuries were awarded only when a physical injury had also occurred.

A criminal offense is the commission of an act forbidden by law, or the omission of an act required by law. Crimes are considered offenses against the state and/or the public welfare and are prosecuted by the state. Among the criminal offenses that have occurred in the delivery of health care are manslaughter, sexual assault and battery, rape, and statutory offenses such as improperly prescribing narcotics.

In recent years, the increasing incidence of child abuse and neglect, abuse of the elderly and dependent adults, and spousal abuse has become more apparent. Indeed, in the early 1990s, domestic violence has captured the attention of federal, state, and local governments, as well as the general population. The trials of Lorena Bobbit, the Menendez brothers, and O.J. Simpson have been covered nationwide; the problem cannot be ignored.

When you have finished reading this chapter, complete the corresponding chapter in your workbook and then go on to Chapter Nine.

REFERENCES

1. Hirsch HL. Outrage gains in suits against MDs. *Legal Aspects of Medical Practice.* November 1979;7:41.
2. Dolan M. High court toughens state fetal murder law. *San Jose Mercury News.* May 17, 1994.
3. Creighton H. *Law Every Nurse Should Know.* 5th ed. Philadelphia, Pa: W.B. Saunders Co.; 1986:231.
4. Balasa DA. Reporting suspected child abuse isn't an option, it's the law! *PMA.* May/June 1992;25:26.
5. My staffers were like family—but one was a thief. *Medical Economics.* December 13, 1993;70:75. Anonymous firsthand account.

9

Public Duties and Responsibilities

In addition to their obligations to individual patients, health care providers have obligations to the states and communities in which they practice. Many of these duties are established by a body of statutes collectively referred to as public health statutes. The purpose of these statutes is to protect the overall health and well-being of the community. Other legislation on subjects ranging from procedures for the involuntary commitment of mental patients to deaths which fall under the jurisdiction of the county medical examiner create additional obligations for health care providers. In addition to conforming to state statutes, health care professionals must also conform to federal statutes— for example, the Controlled Substances Act of 1970.

OBJECTIVES

After studying this chapter, you will be able to:

1. Give two examples of vital statistics reports.
2. State the health care provider's reporting responsibilities in each of the following situations:

   a. Attending a home birth.
   b. Attending a patient whose death occurs as a result of natural causes.
   c. Attending a birth which occurs in a hospital.

3. Briefly describe the types of drugs sought to be controlled by the Controlled Substances Act and give three examples.
4. List two record keeping requirements of the Controlled Substances Act.
5. State the primary purposes of the Controlled Substances Act of 1970.

6. Explain the procedures for chain of custody and chain of evidence.

PUBLIC HEALTH STATUTES AND REQUIRED REPORTS

Public health laws vary from state to state, but they have several common features and goals. These include provisions for:

- Ensuring sanitary conditions in public places.
- Inspecting establishments in which food and drink are processed and sold.
- Exterminating vermin and other pests.
- Monitoring water quality.
- Establishing control measures for certain types of diseases.
- Requiring certain health reports from doctors, school nurses, and other health workers.

It is in the area of required reports that public health statutes most often affect health care professionals. In reading the following summary of these required reports, keep in mind that the health care professional's obligation to comply with the law supersedes his/her obligation to keep patient information confidential.

Vital Statistics

All states collect vital statistics on their citizens. Vital statistics is the broad term covering birth, marriage, divorce, and death records.

Births

The form of live birth certificate varies somewhat among the states, but most utilize the United States Standard Certificate of Live Birth or a similar form (See Figure 9-A).

Figure 9-A. U.S. Standard Certificate of Live Birth

Source: Physicians' Handbook on Medical Certification of Death.
*Hyattsville, MD: National Center for Health Statistics, 1994:5.V.S.U.S.
Dept. of Health and Human Services. PHS 4-1406*

The standard form consists of two parts. The upper portion contains: the name and sex of the child; the date, time, and place of birth; the names, ages, and address(es) of the parents; and the name and signature of the professional person attending the birth (usually a doctor but sometimes a nurse midwife or other health professional) who certifies that the event occurred. The data found in this upper part of the certificate is usually what is furnished by the state when someone requests a copy of his/her birth certificate.

The lower portion of the typical birth certificate contains information collected strictly for medical, health, research, or social purposes. This data is not routinely provided in requests for copies of birth certificates. Information sought includes: the race and educational backgrounds of the parents; medical and health information relating to the mother's pregnancy, labor, and delivery; and information concerning the newborn's medical and health status. The doctor attending a birth is the source of medical information requested in the form. The remaining information requested is usually provided by the mother or father.

When a birth occurs in a hospital, a hospital official sees that the information requested in the certificate is collected and filed with the proper state agency. The doctor attending the birth is responsible for certifying that the event occurred, and for verifying the accuracy of the medical information found in the certificate.

When a birth occurs at home, the attending doctor is responsible for collecting the information and filing the birth certificate. In the absence of a doctor, the nurse midwife, mother, father, or other person in charge of the birth should assume this responsibility.

Deaths

A body must never be disposed of until a doctor has completed the medical portion of a death certificate, signed it, and transmitted it to the funeral director in charge of the funeral arrangements. Under usual circumstances, and when the death is due to natural causes, the doctor attending the patient at the time of death must assume the foregoing responsibilities. However, doctors are also responsible for knowing state and local regulations governing those cases that must be reported to medical examiners and/or coroners.

The U.S. Standard Certificate of Death (Figure 9-B) or a similar form is used by most states.

Figure 9-B. U.S. Standard Certificate of Death

U.S. STANDARD CERTIFICATE OF DEATH

LOCAL FILE NUMBER | STATE FILE NUMBER

1. DECEDENT'S NAME (First, Middle, Last): John Leonard Palmer
2. SEX: Male
3. DATE OF DEATH (Month, Day, Year): June 20, 1989
4. SOCIAL SECURITY NUMBER: 123-45-6789
5a. AGE—Last Birthday (Years): 78
5b. UNDER 1 YEAR (Months, Days)
5c. UNDER 1 DAY (Hours, Minutes)
6. DATE OF BIRTH (Month, Day, Year): April 23, 1911
7. BIRTHPLACE (City and State or Foreign Country): San Francisco, CA
8. WAS DECEDENT EVER IN U.S. ARMED FORCES? (Yes or no): Yes
8a. PLACE OF DEATH (Check only one; see instructions on other side): HOSPITAL ☒ Inpatient ☐ ER Outpatient ☐ DOA — OTHER ☐ Nursing Home ☐ Residence ☐ Other (Specify)
9b. FACILITY NAME (If not institution, give street and number): Mountain Memorial Hospital
9c. CITY, TOWN, OR LOCATION OF DEATH: Frederick
9d. COUNTY OF DEATH: Frederick
10. MARITAL STATUS - Married, Never Married, Widowed, Divorced (Specify): Married
11. SURVIVING SPOUSE (If wife, give maiden name): Sheila Marie Sonner
12a. DECEDENT'S USUAL OCCUPATION (Give kind of work done during most of working life. Do not use retired.): Certified Public Accountant
12b. KIND OF BUSINESS/INDUSTRY: Self-employed
13a. RESIDENCE STATE: Maryland
13b. COUNTY: Frederick
13c. CITY, TOWN, OR LOCATION: Thurmont
13d. STREET AND NUMBER: 245 Lone View Road
13e. INSIDE CITY LIMITS? (Yes or no): No
13f. ZIP CODE: 20212
14. WAS DECEDENT OF HISPANIC ORIGIN? (Specify No or Yes. If yes, specify Cuban, Mexican, Puerto Rican, etc.): No ☒
15. RACE—American Indian, Black, White, etc (Specify): White
16. DECEDENT'S EDUCATION (Specify only highest grade completed) Elementary/Secondary (0-12) College (1-4 or 5+): 4
17. FATHER'S NAME (First, Middle, Last): Stanley Leonard Palmer
18. MOTHER'S NAME (First, Middle, Maiden Surname): Lorraine Ellen Russell
19a. INFORMANT'S NAME (Type/Print): Sheila Marie Palmer
19b. MAILING ADDRESS (Street and Number or Rural Route Number, City or Town, State, Zip Code): 245 Lone View Road, Thurmont, MD 20212
20a. METHOD OF DISPOSITION: ☒ Burial ☐ Cremation ☐ Removal from State ☐ Donation ☐ Other (Specify)
20b. PLACE OF DISPOSITION (Name of cemetery, crematory, or other place): Wesley Memorial Cemetery
20c. LOCATION—City or Town, State: Frederick, MD
21a. SIGNATURE OF FUNERAL SERVICE LICENSEE OR PERSON ACTING AS SUCH: Robert G. Boone
21b. LICENSE NUMBER (of Licensee): 2569114
22. NAME AND ADDRESS OF FACILITY: Boone and Sons Funeral Home 475 E. Main St., Frederick, MD 20216
23a. To the best of my knowledge, death occurred at the time, date, and place stated. Signature and Title: Julia R. Kovar, M.D.
23b. LICENSE NUMBER: 624998075
23c. DATE SIGNED (Month, Day, Year): June 20, 1989
24. TIME OF DEATH: 3:05 AM
25. DATE PRONOUNCED DEAD (Month, Day, Year): June 20, 1989
26. WAS CASE REFERRED TO MEDICAL EXAMINER/CORONER? (Yes or no): No

27. PART I. Enter the diseases, injuries, or complications that caused the death. Do not enter the mode of dying, such as cardiac or respiratory arrest, shock, or heart failure. List only one cause on each line.

Approximate Interval Between Onset and Death

IMMEDIATE CAUSE (Final disease or condition resulting in death) → a. Pulmonary Embolism — Minutes
DUE TO (OR AS A CONSEQUENCE OF): b. Congestive Heart Failure — 4 days
Sequentially list conditions, if any, leading to immediate cause. Enter UNDERLYING CAUSE (Disease or injury that initiated events resulting in death) LAST — DUE TO (OR AS A CONSEQUENCE OF): c. Acute Myocardial Infarction — 7 days
DUE TO (OR AS A CONSEQUENCE OF): d. Chronic Ischemic Heart Disease — 8 years

PART II. Other significant conditions contributing to death but not resulting in the underlying cause given in Part I: Diabetes mellitus, Hypertension

28a. WAS AN AUTOPSY PERFORMED? (Yes or no): No
28b. WERE AUTOPSY FINDINGS AVAILABLE PRIOR TO COMPLETION OF CAUSE OF DEATH? (Yes or no)

29. MANNER OF DEATH: ☒ Natural ☐ Pending Investigation ☐ Accident ☐ Suicide ☐ Could not be Determined ☐ Homicide
30a. DATE OF INJURY (Month, Day, Year)
30b. TIME OF INJURY
30c. INJURY AT WORK? (Yes or no)
30d. DESCRIBE HOW INJURY OCCURRED
30e. PLACE OF INJURY—At home, farm, street, factory, office building, etc. (Specify)
30f. LOCATION (Street and Number or Rural Route Number, City or Town, State)

31a. CERTIFIER (Check only one):
☒ CERTIFYING PHYSICIAN (Physician certifying cause of death when another physician has pronounced death and completed item 23) To the best of my knowledge, death occurred due to the cause(s) and manner as stated.
☐ PRONOUNCING AND CERTIFYING PHYSICIAN (Physician both pronouncing death and certifying to cause of death) To the best of my knowledge, death occurred at the time, date, and place, and due to the cause(s) and manner as stated.
☐ MEDICAL EXAMINER/CORONER On the basis of examination and/or investigation, in my opinion, death occurred at the time, date, and place, and due to the cause(s) and manner as stated.
31b. SIGNATURE AND TITLE OF CERTIFIER: Edmund M. Stone, M.D.
31c. LICENSE NUMBER: 1299654
31d. DATE SIGNED (Month, Day, Year): June 22, 1989
32. NAME AND ADDRESS OF PERSON WHO COMPLETED CAUSE OF DEATH ITEM 27) (Type/Print): Edmund Matthew Stone, M.D. 23 Porter Drive Frederick, MD 29885
33. REGISTRAR'S SIGNATURE: Lori T. Burrette
34. DATE FILED (Month, Day, Year): June 23, 1989

PHS-T-003 REV. 1/89

Left margin: TYPE/PRINT IN PERMANENT BLACK INK FOR INSTRUCTIONS SEE OTHER SIDE AND HANDBOOK — DECEDENT — NAME OF DECEDENT: J. LENARD PALMER For use by physician or institution — SEE INSTRUCTIONS ON OTHER SIDE — PARENTS — INFORMANT — 1989 REVISION — DISPOSITION — SEE DEFINITION ON OTHER SIDE — PRONOUNCING PHYSICIAN ONLY — ITEMS 24-26 MUST BE COMPLETED BY PERSON WHO PRONOUNCES DEATH — SEE INSTRUCTIONS ON OTHER SIDE — CAUSE OF DEATH — SEE DEFINITION ON OTHER SIDE — CERTIFIER — NATIONAL CENTER FOR HEALTH STATISTICS PUBLIC HEALTH SERVICE DEPARTMENT OF HEALTH AND HUMAN SERVICES

Physicians' Handbook on Medical Certification of Death. *Hyattsville, MD: National Center for Health Statistics, 1994:5.V.S.U.S. Dept. of Health and Human Services. PHS 4-1406*

The top half of this form is usually completed by the funeral director. If the death occurred in a hospital it may be completed by hospital personnel Before the body is disposed of, the deceased's attending doctor or a medical examiner completes the lower half and forwards it to the funeral director, who files it with the proper state registrar.

Stillbirths

A special fetal death certificate combining the relevant features of birth and death certificates has been adopted in many states (See Figure 9-C, U.S. Standard Report of Fetal Death). In the absence of a stillbirth certificate, both birth and death certificates may have to be filed.

Preparing Certificates

All vital statistics reports and certificates should be prepared as permanent records. The National Center for Health Statistics recommends the following:

- File the original certificate or report with the registrar. Reproductions or duplicates are not acceptable.
- Avoid abbreviations except those recommended in the specific item instructions.
- Verify with the informant the spelling of names, especially those that have different spellings for the same sound (Smith or Smyth, Gail or Gayle, Wolf or Wolfe, and so forth).
- Refer problems not covered in these instructions to the state office of vital statistics or to the local registrar.
- Use the current form designated by the state.
- Type all entries whenever possible. If a typewriter cannot be used, print legibly in permanent black ink.
- Complete each item, following the specific instructions for that item.
- Do not make alterations or erasures.

- Obtain all signatures; rubber stamps or other facsimile signatures are not acceptable.[1]

Figure 9-C. U.S. Standard Report of Fetal Death

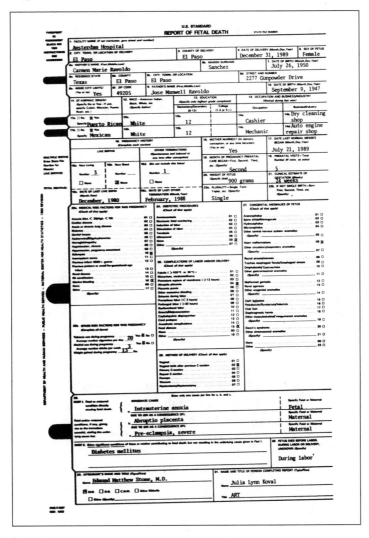

Source: Physicians' Handbook on Medical Certification of Death.
Hyattsville, MD: National Center for Health Statistics, 1994:5.V.S.U.S.
Dept. of Health and Human Services. PHS 4-1406

Autopsies and Reports to Medical Examiners

The county medical examiner or coroner (if a doctor) identifies homicides, suicides, accidental deaths, and sudden deaths due to natural causes.

In all states, the medical examiner has jurisdiction over any case in which a criminal or violent act is a suspected cause of death. Most states also give the medical examiner jurisdiction over any deaths in which the:

- Cause is unknown.
- Deceased was not attended by a doctor at the time of death or for a reasonable amount of time preceding the death.
- Attending doctor was unable to establish a diagnosis before the patient died.

Whenever a case comes under the jurisdiction of the medical examiner, he/she is responsible for executing the medical portion of the death certificate. He/she also has the authority to order and/or perform an autopsy on the body.

The patient's right to noninterference with his/her body—a subject that is discussed throughout this book—does not cease upon his/her death; rather it passes to his/her spouse or next of kin. This person has a property right to the body for the purpose of burying it. Unless a death falls within the jurisdiction of a county medical examiner, an autopsy may never be performed without the valid consent of the person with first right to the body. Violating this right may subject the offender to a civil suit and/or to criminal prosecution.

> A 16-year-old boy suffering from Marfan's disease died in his sleep at boarding school. There were no external signs of the cause of death, so the medical examiner performed an autopsy. The cause of death was discovered to be the effects of Marfan's. The boy's mother sued for an unauthorized autopsy, but the court dismissed her suit because state law permitted an autopsy without consent when the cause of death was "obscure." (*Donnelly v Guion*, 467 F.2d 290, 1972)

Infectious, Contagious, or Communicable Diseases Reports

To protect the general health and welfare of their citizens, all states require the reporting of certain diseases to the county or state health department. State regulations specifically charge doctors with this reporting responsibility, but the regulations also contain the statement that *anyone* with knowledge of a suspected or confirmed case of a reportable disease must make the report. Individual state regulations stipulate how quickly the report must be made and through what communications medium (e.g., telephone or mail).

Every medical office should have reference information on reportable diseases and reporting regulations. A supply of case report forms (Figure 9-D) should also be maintained. These materials are available through the appropriate county or state health department.

Figure 9-D. Communicable Disease Report Form

Source: Illinois Department of Public Health. Used with permission.

Failure to Report

Failure to file a report that is required by statute may result in criminal prosecution by the state; if someone is damaged, the result may be a civil suit by a private party.

Other Reportable Conditions

Some states require that **cancer** detections be reported to health officials so that the state can monitor the disease and help identify environmental causes.

Recent advancements now enable doctors to identify and treat several potentially severe **congenital disorders** in newborn babies. Since early detection is critical to successful treatment, many state statutes and/or health department regulations require that newborns be tested for congenital hypothyroidism, phenylketonuria (PKU), and galactosemia. These **metabolic disorders** can cause serious physical and mental problems if not properly and promptly treated.

The testing is usually done within three days of birth. Positive results are reported to a local health department official, who is responsible for follow-up action. For hospital births, the responsibility for performing the tests is either that of hospital personnel or the attending doctor. For home births, the doctor, nurse midwife, or person in charge is responsible for seeing that the infant is properly tested.

Some states require doctors to report diseases that may cause a lapse of consciousness, such as **epilepsy**. The report is sent to the state motor vehicle division to determine a person's eligibility to drive on public roads.

In some states, cases of suspected or confirmed **pesticide poisoning** must be reported in some states. Information is relayed from the health department to other state agencies, which investigate the case.

Injuries Caused by Acts of Violence

All states require doctors to report immediately to local law enforcement agencies any injury whose known or suspected cause is a violent act. The doctor may treat the patient for the injury, but a telephone report must be made immediately thereafter so that the proper authorities may investigate the situation. The report should include the patient's name, whereabouts, and extent of injuries.

Chain of Custody of Specimens

When specimens are obtained that might be significant in a legal situation or a court case, the chain of custody of those specimens is of critical importance. If the procedure is not properly followed or the paperwork is inaccurate or incomplete, the validity of the specimens is compromised.

The chain of custody form is used to ensure the integrity of the specimen and to verify that the specimen was handled properly. The responsibilities of laboratory and office personnel include the following:

1. Observe the actual collection of the specimen from the patient.
2. Completely and accurately label the specimen and complete, sign, and date the form.
3. Obtain the patient's initials on the form to indicate his/her verification of the specimen's authenticity.
4. Place the top copy of the form in the clear plastic bag with the specimen. Make sure the patient's name is visible and seal the bag. If the name is not visible, the bag would have to be opened, thus invalidating the chain of custody.
5. Attach the first copy to the bag. It is signed by each person who handles the specimen. Place the second copy in the office or laboratory file.

Chain of Evidence

Generally, the collection of evidence of a crime resulting in the injury of the victim would be undertaken by emergency room or hospital personnel. There may be occasions, however, when the victim of a crime might be seen in the office setting. In such a case, it is necessary to obtain, preserve, and protect the integrity of possible evidence.

Careful, complete documentation in the patient record is the type of evidence most frequently used in civil and criminal cases. Evidence in criminal cases might include photos; x-rays; blood specimens, tissue, semen, vomitus, or other bodily fluids; foreign objects such as bullets, gravel, bits of metal; hair or nail clippings; and clothing. All specimens must be carefully obtained and preserved in sealed bags, if possible. Complete identification must be placed with the piece of evidence. All forms of evidence must be held in a locked cabinet until delivered to the proper authorities and a receipt received. To maintain integrity and validity, only one member of the staff should handle evidence.

Evidence should be handled as little as possible. Photos should be taken as soon as possible and, if possible, before clothing is removed. If the removal of clothing requires that it be cut, it should be done so along seams and away from evidence of the crime (e.g., bullet holes, tears, or vomitus). Should the patient die in the office, the body should not be touched nor any possible evidence removed.

COMPETENCY CHECK: ONE

1. What are a doctor's responsibilities with regard to completing the death certificate on a patient who has died due to natural causes?

2. Most states give medical examiners jurisdiction over cases when the death was the result of one of three causes. Name them.

3. Why do states require doctors to report the occurrence of certain communicable diseases?

4. True or false: Health care personnel may be responsible for preserving evidence of a crime.

Commitment of the Mentally Ill

Procedures for the detention and commitment of mentally ill persons are subjects of study, concern, and debate for both the medical and legal professions. Some people believe that mental illness is strictly a health problem, and therefore the decision for commitment should be made solely by doctors. Others believe that since commitment deprives people of their basic legal rights, the decision to commit a person should be made by the courts. Since voluntary commitments do not pose the same legal problems as involuntary commitments, our attention will focus on involuntary commitment procedures. State laws vary, but the following requirements appear in most statutes:

- A patient should be urged to commit himself/herself voluntarily before involuntary commitment procedures are initiated.
- Hospitalization may be authorized only when there is recent, direct evidence that a person may be harmful to himself/herself or others.
- A doctor must certify to the need for commitment, and the certification must be based on a valid and recent medical examination.
- The patient must be notified in advance that he/she is to be committed, and why this must be done. In some cases, a close relative must also be notified.
- A formal hearing must be conducted on the need for the commitment, with the decision being made by a judge, jury, or special committee.
- The patient may have the assistance of legal counsel at relevant times.

Doctors are responsible for knowing and abiding by the statutes governing commitment procedures in their states. As pointed out in an earlier chapter, failure to abide by statutory regulations constitutes the tort of false imprisonment. Certifying that a patient has been examined and found to be in need of compulsory hospitalization, when in fact the doctor never examined the patient, is a statutory violation severely punished by most courts.

Care of the mentally ill continues to be one of the most challenging medicolegal problems. Among the issues that must be addressed is whether the patient has the right to:

- Adequate treatment, or custodial care.
- A timely discharge, or a discharge worked out as soon as staff and court system permit.
- Be free of mechanical restraints.
- Communicate freely with relatives, including the right to send and receive uncensored mail, and to have visitors at his/her convenience.
- Refuse therapeutic treatment.

CONTROLLED SUBSTANCES ACT OF 1970

We have seen that most laws affecting the practice of medicine and the delivery of health care originate within each of the fifty states. Licenses to practice, legal remedies for civil offenses, statutes of limitations, and misdeeds constituting torts or criminal offenses are all matters addressed and determined by state legislatures and state courts.

One area of health care is regulated primarily by federal law: the prescribing, administering, and dispensing of drugs classified as controlled substances. Controlled substances are narcotics and other dangerous drugs that can easily be abused, causing the user to become psychologically and/or physically dependent.

The drug abuse problem has always been a serious one, but the extent of the problem increased in the 1960s. During that decade, it became apparent that stricter control of certain drugs was necessary to stop their diversion from legitimate medical purposes to illegal purposes. The goal of additional control was to prevent those people who were illegally using drugs from obtaining them. To create a closed system of legitimate distribution, controls had to be imposed at the federal level.

In the fall of 1970, a new federal drug law was enacted. Frequently referred to as the Controlled Substances Act, its official title is the Comprehensive Drug Abuse Prevention and Control Act of 1970. A federal agency called the Bureau of Narcotics and Dangerous Drugs (BNDD), an agency within the Department of Justice, was given responsibility for enforcing this law.

In 1973, after several name changes due to reorganization, the BNDD was renamed the Drug Enforcement Administration (DEA). The agency is still within the Department of Justice and is still accountable to the United States Attorney General.

The Controlled Substances Act of 1970 is a very broad statute that replaced many federal laws regulating narcotics and other dangerous drugs. In replacing these laws, it consolidated and tightened federal control over the manufacture, distribution, and dispensing of drugs considered to have a high potential for abuse. The act imposes jurisdiction over "every person who manufactures, distributes, or dispenses any controlled substance." While the scope and depth of this comprehensive and complex law cannot be covered here, those provisions of direct and immediate concern to health care professionals are included.

Classification of Controlled Substances

The law classifies the drugs it wishes to control into five schedules, Schedules I through V. The criteria for classifying a drug are stated in the statute, and specific drugs are listed within each schedule. Each schedule is regulated independently and according to the degree of control sought over the drugs listed within the schedule. The following schedule summaries illustrate this aspect of the law.

Schedule I

These substances have high potential for abuse and no accepted medical use. Even under medical supervision, Schedule I substances are considered unsafe. These substances are of interest and value only to research doctors and may not be prescribed by practicing physicians. Examples include heroin, LSD, and peyote.

Schedule II

While these drugs also have a high potential for abuse, they have accepted medical uses. Schedule II substances are the most closely regulated. To obtain a supply for office or medical bag use, the physician must use special triplicate order forms available only through the DEA. In addition, many states require that prescriptions for Schedule II narcotics be written on special prescription blanks available through the state department of health or justice. The prescription must be handwritten by the physician in ink or indelible pen, and it may not be refilled. Only in the case of a genuine emergency may a pharmacist accept an oral prescription for a Schedule II drug, and only the amount necessary to cope with the emergency will be provided. The physician must submit to the pharmacist a written, signed prescription within seventy-two hours. If the physician fails to do so, the pharmacist must notify the DEA. Examples of Schedule II substances include: codeine, morphine, opium, and amphetamines.

Schedule III

These substances have less potential for abuse than those listed in Schedule II, and they have many accepted medical uses. Abuse may lead to moderate or low physical dependence or high psychological dependence. Prescriptions for Schedule III substances may be oral or written and, if authorized by the prescribing physician, refilled a maximum of five times within a six-month period. These drugs include compounds of narcotic and non-narcotic substances, central nervous system stimulants, some depressants, and short-acting barbiturates. Examples include Tylenol or Empirin compound with codeine, Doriden, and paregoric.

Schedule IV

These substances have less potential for abuse than those in Schedule III and have many accepted medical uses. The longer-acting barbiturates, some tranquilizers, and antidepressants are included here. Prescriptions may be refilled a maximum of five times within a five-month period. Specific examples include chloral hydrate, Equanil, Librium, and phenobarbital.

Schedule V

These substances have an abuse potential less than those listed in Schedule IV and include preparations with a very small amount of certain narcotics. Many of these are available without a prescription, such as cough syrup with codeine.

COMPETENCY CHECK: TWO

5. **What is the primary goal of the Controlled Substances Act of 1970?**

6. **Which schedule of drugs is the most closely regulated and why?**

Before studying additional provisions of the Controlled Substances Act, the terms administer, dispense, and prescribe should be clearly understood, as well as the differences between them:

- To **administer** a drug is to place it directly in the patient's body, such as through an injection.
- To **dispense** a drug is to give it to the patient in a container for later use.
- To **prescribe** a drug is to write an order for a drug, with the order to be filled by a pharmacist, who actually dispenses the drug.

Registration

Any doctor who administers, prescribes, or dispenses any scheduled drug must first register with the Drug Enforcement Administration (DEA). The registration number assigned by that agency is required to appear on all prescriptions for controlled substances, and the registration must be renewed annually.

If a doctor administers or dispenses controlled substances through more than one office, he/she must register each office and must obtain a registration number for use at each. If he/she administers or dispenses only at his/her principal office and merely prescribes at the other(s), he/she need register only the principal office. Any change in office address must be reported to the DEA.

A doctor who dispenses or intends to dispense narcotics as maintenance dosages or as part of detoxification treatment must obtain a special registration permit from the DEA.

A doctor who regularly dispenses controlled substances must take a written inventory of his/her drug supply every two years and keep the record an additional two years. The DEA may inspect it at any time.

Record Keeping

A doctor who dispenses any narcotic drugs must keep a
special record showing each transaction. A doctor who
routinely dispenses and charges patients for non-narcotic
controlled substances must keep a special record of all
transactions. A doctor who occasionally dispenses a non-
narcotic controlled substance in the form of a doctor's
sample does not have to make a special record of the transaction, except for the usual notation in the patient's chart.

Dispensing records of controlled substances must be
kept for two years and are subject to inspection by the
DEA. Required information includes the full name and
address of the patient, the date the drug was given, the
quantity and character of the drug, and how it was dispensed. It is suggested that a special book be maintained for
recording transactions involving controlled substances.
Many medical office supply houses have record books and
forms especially designed for keeping dispensing records.

Upon retirement or discontinuation of practice, a doctor
must return to the DEA his/her registration certificate and
any unused order forms for Schedule II substances. Any
controlled substances on hand at the time of the office closing should be disposed of according to DEA instructions.

Controlled substances kept in doctors' offices must be
stored in solidly constructed, locked safes or cabinets.
Thefts must be reported immediately to the closest regional
DEA office and the local police.

Violating any provision of the Controlled Substances
Act is a criminal offense. Penalties range from small fines
for less serious violations to lengthy jail sentences and large
fines for more serious offenses. The charges brought and
penalties imposed usually depend on the provision violated,
whether criminal intent was involved, and whether the violation was a first or a repeat offense. Recall that conviction
of a crime often results in the doctor's license being suspended or revoked.

An elderly physician opened and operated a rural clinic after
retiring from a general surgery practice. Most of his clinic

patients were overweight and sought help for that reason. Treatment consisted of a very brief physical examination, a lecture and pamphlet on weight control, and the dispensing of certain controlled drugs. He was charged with twenty-five counts of dispensing and distributing controlled substances not in good faith or for legitimate medical purposes. The charges were brought by six undercover DEA agents who posed as patients for ten months. The physician was found guilty on all counts. (*U.S. v Rosen*, 448 F.S.926, 1977)

State Laws Regarding Controlled Substances

Since the passage of the Controlled Substances Act of 1970, most states have enacted legislation that conforms to and complements the federal law. The common provisions of state laws:

- Require registration by doctors with the designated state agency.
- Stipulate who is authorized to prescribe.
- Specify the form and the required content of written prescriptions for controlled substances.
- Specify circumstances under which oral prescriptions will be filled by pharmacists.
- Establish state record keeping requirements (usually the same as federal requirements).
- Determine how and where addicts and habitual users may be treated for addiction.
- State penalties for violations.

Many states prohibit doctors from self-prescribing or self-administering narcotics. Prescribing controlled substances without a proper medical examination is also an offense in most states, as it is under federal law.

Precautions

To addicts, doctors' offices are logical sources of the drugs needed to sustain their habits. There are a number of precautions medical office personnel can take to prevent controlled substances from falling into the hands of addicts or unauthorized handlers. Many of the following security suggestions have been adapted from ideas presented in *The Medical Assistant*, by Cooper and Cooper.[2]

- While the doctor's bag is in the office, it should be stored in a place inaccessible to any patients. The bag should never be left in a car where it can be seen. If it must be left in a car, it should be stored in a locked trunk.
- Prescription blanks should not be left in unattended places within the office. It is frequently recommended that all prescription pads, especially narcotics forms, be kept under lock and key except for the one currently in use. That one should be kept either in the doctor's desk drawer or on his/her person. Where state regulations require the use of serially-numbered prescription blanks for controlled substances, the pad should be checked periodically to make sure the blanks are in correct sequence. Irregularities should be reported to the doctor; if unexplainable, the doctor will probably want the discrepancy reported to the proper authorities.
- Prescription blanks that have special features to minimize the possibility of alteration or enhance the detection of thefts can be obtained. For example, blanks may be numbered and issued consecutively to facilitate the detection of theft. Having the blanks printed with a special pattern would help the pharmacist detect alterations.

A pharmacist can help prevent controlled substances from falling into the hands of drug addicts or unauthorized handlers by checking with the doctor's office whenever a suspicious prescription is encountered. The health care professional handling such an inquiry should check the patient's record to verify all elements of the prescription.

The health care professional who takes patient histories must be alert for the new patient who, after describing certain symptoms, claims that the only known relief for his/her condition is a particular controlled substance. Self-diagnosis and self-prescribing are often clues that the patient is an addict. Behavior of this type should be reported to the doctor before the patient is seen or treated. As stated earlier, it is a state and federal offense for a doctor to prescribe a controlled substance without physically examining the patient and making an independent diagnosis.

COMPETENCY CHECK: THREE

7. **A physician occasionally dispenses narcotics. What special records must be kept in order to comply with the federal Controlled Substances Act?**

8. **With which federal agency must a doctor register before administering, dispensing, or prescribing any controlled substance?**

9. **List three precautions that should be taken by medical office personnel to prevent access to controlled substances by illegitimate users.**

SUMMARY

In addition to their obligations to individual patients, health care professionals have obligations to the states and communities in which they live, and to the federal government.

Major obligations to the states relate to public health statutes and required reports. Required reports include:

1. Vital statistics (births, deaths, marriages, and divorces), and reports to the medical examiner or coroner concerning deaths due to specific circumstances.
2. Reports to state health officials concerning infectious, contagious, and communicable disease. State requirements vary concerning other reportable conditions. Some states, for example, require the reporting of cancer, congenital metabolic disorders, and epilepsy.

At the federal level, the Controlled Substances Act of 1970 brought about a tighter rein on the manufacture, distribution, dispensing, and use of controlled substances.

Enforced by the Drug Enforcement Administration of the Justice Department, the Controlled Substances Act has specific requirements covering, for example, registration of doctors and record keeping. States also have laws related to controlled substances. Such laws vary by state, but most have basic requirements in common.

Controlled substances and prescription blanks in the doctor's office and car should be safeguarded. Moreover, doctors and other health care professionals should be alert to symptoms of narcotics addiction manifested by their patients.

When you have finished reading this chapter, complete the corresponding chapter in your workbook and then go on to Chapter Ten.

REFERENCES

1. *Physicians Handbook on Medical Certification of Death.* Hyattsville, MD: National Center for Health Statistics; 1994 reprint:5. U.S. Dept. of Health and Human Services (PHS) 4-1046.
2. Cooper MG., Cooper ME. *The Medical Assistant.* 5th ed. St. Louis, Mo: McGraw Hill, 1986:480-488.

10

Patient Health Records

Medical records have scientific, educational, financial, legal, and social purposes. No matter what one's perspective, the importance of patient records cannot be overstated, and almost every chapter in this book includes a direct or indirect reference to them. This chapter will summarize important legal points concerning medical records.

OBJECTIVES

After studying this chapter, you will be able to:

1. List and briefly describe four purposes served by keeping patient records.
2. State who owns hospital, clinic, and office records, and who has a right to the information in them.
3. List five record keeping practices that will enhance the legal value of a patient record.
4. Describe three steps needed to properly correct a patient record entry.
5. State specific steps that a custodian of records should take when served with a *subpoena duces tecum*.

OVERVIEW

Although licensing regulations require hospitals to keep patient records, there are no comparable regulations requiring doctors to keep medical records on patients treated in their offices. Clearly, however, doctors have professional, personal, medical, and legal reasons for doing so. Keeping accurate office records is as essential to the doctor as employing well-qualified health care professionals.

As stated before, medical records have many functions—both practical and legal. In this overview, we will take a general look at the record: its purpose, content, ownership, and retention.

PURPOSES

First, let us look at the purposes and uses of the patient record: an aid to practicing medicine; an aid to communication; a legal document; the basis of peer review; and a tool in medical research and teaching.

An Aid to Practicing Medicine

Patient records provide doctors with the clinical data that enable them to diagnose problems and plan treatment. Over time, a patient's record profiles his/her personal health. It may provide clues to genetic problems, inherited tendencies, and the relationship between past and present problems. Given the patient caseload of most doctors and the amount of laboratory testing and related work, it would be difficult to practice without a record keeping system.

An Aid to Communication

The patient record is a means of communication between doctors and other persons involved in health care delivery. In hospitals, the record is the primary communications link between the attending doctor and other members of the health care team. Doctors write their orders in the records and others execute those orders and record the results of their actions. In office practice, the record is a similar means of communication between doctors and other health care professionals.

The following case tragically illustrates how an unclear record can result in serious miscommunication.

A three-month-old infant had been intermittently hospitalized throughout her short life and was once again admitted. The baby was receiving daily 2.5 c.c.s. of Elixir Pediatric Lanoxin administered orally by her mother according to the physician's instructions. One day the physician increased the dosage to 3.0

c.c.s. and so informed the mother. He made the following notation in the hospital chart: "Give 3.0 c.c.s. Lanoxin today for
one dose only." A temporary nurse, not familiar with the
arrangement worked out between the physician and the baby's
mother, noted the instruction, and finding no indication that the
dose had been administered, injected 3.0 c.c.s. of Lanoxin into
the infant. The overdose caused the infant's death. The physician, nurse, and hospital were all sued: the nurse, because it
was her act that caused the patient's death and because she
failed to question the physician about a dosage she should have
known was too large; the hospital, as the nurse's employer; and
the physician, for his negligent record keeping. (*Norton v
Argonaut Insurance Company,* 144 So.2d 249; La. 1962)

The patient record is also a means of communication
between past and present doctors, and between primary care
doctors and those professionals consulted for special problems or studies.

An elderly patient was admitted to a hospital for a diagnostic
study. Her chief complaints were general fatigue, stomach
pains, and fainting. As her family physician instructed, she was
taken to the radiology department for a series of x-rays. During
one of the procedures, the patient fainted and fell. The fall
caused a fractured hip, the treatment of which caused or aggravated other medical problems. The patient sued the radiologist
and the hospital. The radiologist was found liable for not
acquainting himself with the patient's history, and the hospital
was found negligent for its policy of not requiring a patient's
medical history to be entered on x-ray requisition forms.
(*Favalora v Aetna Casualty and Surety Company,* 144 So.2d
544, La. 1962)

A Legal Document

The ideal patient record is an objective, factual account of a
patient's health history, present condition, and prognosis.
All entries are relevant, significant, and pertinent. This written record often determines whether a lawsuit is filed, the
outcome of a suit that is tried, and the amount of damages
awarded. Because the quality of the medical record often
reflects the quality of care a patient has received, the record
is, as one author has put it, "The doctor's best friend—or
worst enemy." [1]

Basis of Peer Review

Medical audit and peer review committees use medical records to evaluate a doctor's competence. In many hospitals, a doctor will lose hospital privileges for not keeping adequate hospital records or for not completing them promptly.

Use in Patient Research and Teaching

Patient records are an important source of research, teaching, and health care planning. However, patient records may not be used for even these worthwhile purposes without the patient's consent.

CONTENTS

The typical office record consists of two parts: (1) personal information provided by the patient; and (2) clinical information supplied by the doctor or the authorized agent(s).

The personal information section includes the patient's full name, address, telephone number, occupation, employer, date of birth, marital status, number of children, source of referral, insurance information, and other identifying information. It also includes the patient's personal and family medical history and the patient's chief complaints.

The clinical information section typically contains physical examination data, laboratory and x-ray reports, diagnoses, treatments prescribed, hospital discharge summaries, progress notes, and the patient's condition and prognosis upon termination of treatment or of the relationship. Every single entry in this section of the record should contribute to an accurate, objective, material, scientific, chronological, and pertinent account of the patient's condition and how it was treated.

Also filed in the patient's record are consent forms for certain office procedures, authorization forms regarding the release of patient information, correspondence, consultation reports, letters of withdrawal or advice, and other relevant documents. Customarily, the hospital record contains consent forms for procedures performed in the hospital, but if a proposed hospital procedure is explained in the office and the patient gives a verbal "informed consent" there, the explanation and the oral consent (as well as the subsequent written document) should be noted in the office record.

All medical office personnel should adhere to the policies and procedures established by the doctor-employer, and should pursue record keeping responsibilities diligently, vigorously, and promptly. Procrastination is the biggest danger facing medical record keepers, for the task is often tedious, routine, and without obvious reward. There is great reward and satisfaction, however, when the record is reviewed or subpoenaed, and the health care professional can produce with pride and confidence an accurate, complete, clear, and neat record.

To reiterate, patient records must be considered legal documents and maintained as though they may be scrutinized at any moment.

OWNERSHIP

The original patient records developed and maintained during the course of patient treatment belong to the owners of the health care facility in which the treatment was provided. Records developed by a doctor during the course of private office practice belong to the doctor. Records initiated and developed in a hospital belong to the hospital. Records initiated and developed in a clinic belong to the clinic owners. These owners have a property right in the original records.

Patients have legal interests in their medical records. They have the right to see and/or obtain a copy of their records. In fact, the law has evolved to the point that a patient's right to the information in his/her record is as great as the hospital's or doctor's property right to the record itself.

This change in legal philosophy is based on several fundamental axioms:

- Health care providers keep records for the benefit of patients as well as for their own benefit and the benefit of their employers.
- Keeping medical records is part of the contractual obligation between health care provider and patient.
- The health care provider is the custodian of the record, but the patient has the right to have access to the information in the record.
- The patient's right to control his/her body and to give an informed consent entitles him/her to access the medical record concerning his/her body.

The courts have recognized, however, that some patients (generally those with mental or emotional disorders) could be harmed by seeing their medical records. In such cases the societal interest of not divulging all parts of the patient's record may outweigh the patient's right to have access to the information.

The courts have also recognized that persons other than doctor and patient sometimes need to see a patient's record. Hospital personnel involved in caring for the patient need access to the record at the time of treatment. As soon as the need ceases, however, so does the right of access.

In response to debates on the best way of providing patients with useful information from their records, several proposals have been developed. The two concepts most widely supported are referred to as patient-carried records and dual records.

- **Patient-carried records** are generally supported by consumer advocates. Proponents recommend that legislation be enacted to require that "a complete and unexpurgated copy of all medical records . . . be issued routinely and automatically to patients as soon as the services provided are recorded."[2]
- Under the **dual record** proposal, two sets of records would be maintained. One would be the official record including "all personal patient data, social and family history, complaints and symptom

descriptions, test and examination results, diagnoses, prescribed treatment or medication, and billing records."[3] The patient would have a copy of this record. The other record, referred to as the "active working record," would contain more sensitive material and tentative hypotheses for the doctor's own use or for that of other professionals involved in caring for the patient.

RETENTION

The value of a patient's health record certainly does not cease as soon as the patient's need for treatment ceases. For many years, the record may serve all of the purposes discussed earlier in this chapter. It may also provide documentation of the patient's right to certain benefits. As the following example illustrates, a record may be of value decades after it was originally made:

> The attorney of a deceased physician called the Illinois Medical Society to find out how long the physician's patient records should be kept. The director of the society's publications advised the attorney to keep at least the face sheets indefinitely. During the following year, the widow of a patient was able to obtain benefits under the Black Lung Act because first the physician and then the attorney kept the records documenting the physician's treatment of the patient for black lung disease thirty-eight years earlier.[4]

For the doctor's legal protection, all patient records should be kept *at least* until germane statutes of limitations have expired. Because statutes of limitations are extended for so many different reasons, however, it is preferable to keep records indefinitely.

COMPETENCY CHECK: ONE

1. True or false: Medical records are kept solely for the doctor's legal protection.

2. True or false: A doctor owns the patient records developed and maintained while in private practice.

3. True or false: Patients have no right to their own health care records.

4. True or false: Doctors co-own those hospital records concerning patients they have admitted or treated in hospitals.

RECORD KEEPING GUIDELINES

- Since the patient record is a legal document, entries must be made in ink and include the date, necessary information, and signature of the physician.
- The patient record should not contain irrelevant observations, teaching notes, or other entries that are unrelated to the patient's care. The record should never include remarks concerning professional disputes or disagreements.

    The following is an example of an inappropriate entry: "The laboratory refused to draw CBC due to personnel shortage. Spoke to supervisor regarding this issue without success. CBC drawn by myself and sent to lab."

    The appropriate entry would have been: "CBC drawn and sent to the lab."

- Errors in the patient record must be corrected, but they must be corrected properly. Never obliterate or erase an original entry. Draw a single line through the incorrect data, and note in the margin who made the change, when, and why. Then enter the correct information in chronological sequence.

    Many experienced medical office personnel believe the appointment book should be handled in a similar fashion. When a patient cancels, changes, or does not keep an appointment, a single line should be drawn through the original entry in the appointment book and a notation should be made describing what happened.

- Deliberately changing a record to conceal a mistake is very foolish. It is also a criminal offense. It is not unheard of for the defendant in a lawsuit to alter a record after learning of the litigation. Changing a record so that it appears to reflect more favorably on one's actions usually has the opposite result, and often the damage award is much larger than it would have been had the record not been changed.

An obstetrician contracted with a patient to deliver her baby. The patient went into labor and was taken to the hospital, where a nurse called the physician. He asked her to delay the birth until he completed his luncheon engagement. When they were unable to do so, a member of the house staff delivered the baby. Complications arose, resulting in the baby's death. The parents sued for breach of contract. The physician changed the hospital records to indicate that he had attended the delivery. However, the woman's husband, anxiously watching the clock in the reception room, saw the physician arrive at exactly the same time as the birth occurred. Obviously, the records had been falsified, and the jury awarded the parents a very large settlement, much larger than would have been awarded for a breach of contract suit.[5]

Changes in records can usually be detected and analyzed to determine who made the changes and when. The ink, handwriting, and even the paper stock can be analyzed and dated.

A physician learned that a minor treated five years earlier was suing because the physician had not performed a drug sensitivity test. In a deposition the physician claimed he had performed the test and that his office records would verify it. The patient's attorney asked to have the record analyzed, but the physician refused. The attorney began legal action to acquire the record, but the defense decided to settle. The strong impression was left that a scientific analysis of the record would have discredited the physician.[6]

- Office personnel should not make entries in a medical record unless authorized to do so by their doctor-employer. The authorization to do so should be in written form and included in the employee's written job description.
- To protect the patient's privacy and to create an atmosphere in which the patient will feel comfort-

able and be candid, the patient's medical history should be taken in private. This sometimes poses problems for office personnel authorized to take histories. Friends or relatives should not be present during the patient's history interview or physical examination unless needed for aiding communication or for medical purposes. In the absence of legitimate need, the health care professional taking the history should tactfully but firmly insist that a friend or relative wait in the reception area.

- Personal opinions, especially derogatory remarks, concerning a patient should not be entered in a medical record. Such remarks do not reflect favorably on professional people trained to be objective helpers. Furthermore, opinionated remarks are difficult to defend on a witness stand.

- While it is common practice among some doctors and other health care professionals to omit notations of negative or normal findings, under scrutiny the omission always poses the question: Were the findings normal or was the test or procedure not performed? When, in hindsight, the results of a test or procedure are crucial to a patient's legal claim, the omitted information may subtly suggest negligence or carelessness. Fairly or not, juries seem to be inclined to conclude the worst. Under any circumstances, failure to note negative or normal findings suggests lazy record keeping.

- To ensure the authenticity of the record as a legal document, entries should be made as the events occur or immediately thereafter. It would be difficult to defend the practice of entering data days after the event transpired. Even if a doctor could recall a patient's blood pressure days after the fact, an opposing trial attorney could raise questions in the jurors' minds about the doctor's ability to do so.

- The following information should always be entered in a record, along with the date and initials of the person making the entry:

1. Notation of missed appointment and action taken.
2. Notation of telephone inquiries of a medical nature, along with advice given.
3. Instructions regarding home care, special diet, weight control, personal habits, physical exercise, etc. Special instructions, such as not mixing certain drugs or not driving while taking a certain medication, should be noted prominently in the record. At appropriate intervals, the patient's degree of cooperation should be noted.
4. Prescription refills.

- On a few occasions, third-party insurance companies have refused to pay claims for services that could not be substantiated in a patient's medical record. To prevent this problem, along with more serious ones, the record keeper should periodically review the records to assess their quality. This review should occur automatically as the record keeper prepares the chart for the patient's appointment, and as the chart is refiled after the patient's visit. The record keeper should check to make sure that test results are recorded as ordered, that procedures are documented, that entries are clearly identified, and that all reports are present and accounted for.
- All entries should be legible and self-explanatory to another doctor or health care professional. Abbreviations or shortened medical terms should be used only when standardized throughout the profession. If unusual short forms of certain words or procedures are used (not a recommended practice), a key to the abbreviations should appear in the chart.
- Information regarding the doctor's fees and the patient's payments should not be intermingled with the medical record. When the medical record is transferred or released to another party, it should not contain financial information.

5. A new patient, a 19-year-old girl, is accompanied to the office by a girlfriend. When the podiatry assistant asks the new patient to come into her office for an interview, the friend follows. What, if any, action should the assistant take?

6. A medical assistant records a blood pressure reading on the wrong chart. How should the error be corrected?

7. Why should negative and normal findings always be noted?

RELEASE OF INFORMATION

A point emphasized throughout this book is that, unless a disclosure is legally required, a patient has the sole authority to release information from his/her medical record. However, a patient's authorization to release information does not mean that the original record or portions of it should be sent to the designated recipient. When the patient authorizes release of information to an insurance company, for example, it is the usual practice for the doctor and the office personnel to complete a claim form based on the medical information contained in the record. In short, the information is released, but not the record itself.

Transfer of Records

Often patients ask their doctors to send their records to another doctor. A doctor may elect to send the entire record, but it is customary to send either a written summary in letter form or a photocopied excerpt from pages of the record that illustrate the patient's relevant history and present condition. If the entire record must be transmitted, it should be photocopied and the copy sent. Sending original records, unless legally required, is not a recommended practice.

Remember that it is the patient's right to have records released or shared, and the doctor or any other health care professional may not negate his/her wishes without legitimate cause. The fact that a patient has not paid a bill does not affect this right. Office personnel often ask if they may refuse to release a record until the patient has paid a bill, and the answer is a definite no. Withholding a patient's records for this reason may subject the doctor and the employee to a civil suit.

Subpoena Duces Tecum

A *subpoena duces tecum* is a court order to appear in a particular court with certain records. Usually the subpoenaed records are a patient's health records, although the doctor's business records may be subpoenaed as well. A patient's records may be subpoenaed for any number of purposes, but the underlying reason is always to acquire written evidence of the patient's condition and of the care received. Given the legal climate today, a health care professional in charge of patient records can count on being served with a *subpoena duces tecum* sooner or later in her/his professional career. The exact nature of her/his response to the subpoena is a matter for her/his doctor-employer and attorney to decide, but the following procedures describe usual practices. The prime objective of these practices is to protect and preserve the integrity of the subpoenaed records:

- After being served with a subpoena by an official court representative, but before the server leaves the premises, the health care professional should:

   1. Check to make sure the name and phone number of the issuing attorney and the court docket number of the case appear on the subpoena.
   2. Verify, if given a photocopy, that it is an exact duplicate of the original held by the server.
   3. Make sure the patient referred to in the subpoena was actually seen by the doctor.

- The doctor should be notified as soon as possible that a *subpoena duces tecum* has been received. Depending on the reason for the subpoena, the doctor's attorney may need to be notified.

- The health care professional should check with the court to make sure the case is scheduled for trial at the time designated in the subpoena.
- The health care professional should review the subpoenaed records to make sure they are complete. Missing reports should be located and inserted. The contents of the medical record, however, should never be altered. Attempts to improve legibility should not be made because they could be construed as attempts to change the record. Items of a nonmedical nature should be removed, however, unless the items were specifically cited in the subpoena.
- The health care professional should number the pages in the record in ink, enter the total number of pages in the file folder, and prepare a cover sheet, in duplicate, that itemizes the contents of the record.
- The record should be stored in a locked office safe for maximum protection.
- If state law and the attorneys involved permit, a photocopy of the original record may be submitted in place of the original. From the doctor's point of view, this is preferable because the original record would not have to leave the office. If the court is willing to accept a photocopy, either or both of the following steps may have to be taken:

1. The health care professional may have to sign a sworn statement that the photocopy is a faithful reproduction of the original record.
2. He/she may have to take both the original record and the photocopy to court, where a court-appointed officer will compare the two to make sure the copy is an exact duplicate.

- If a health care professional must take the record to court himself/herself, he/she must not give or show the record to anyone until instructed to do so

by the judge. Neither should the health care professional leave the record in the possession of anyone
except the judge. Furthermore, he/she should obtain
an official receipt for the record once it is left.

● If a health care professional is required to intro-
duce the records into evidence, he/she will have to
take the stand and be sworn in. He/she could be
questioned about the record or asked to read certain
parts of it, but usually he/she will be asked simply
to submit it and then will be excused from the stand
and the court.

The costs of reproducing subpoenaed records and trans-
porting them to court are borne by the attorney subpoenaing
them. Microfilmed records are normally acceptable as legal
evidence but require special treatment because they contain
information on more than one patient. If a subpoenaed
record is available only on microfilm or microfiche, the
health care professional should so inform the attorney who
subpoenaed it before taking the film to court. The attorney
may decide the record is not necessary in view of the
expense of having it read or reproduced. Under no circumstances should the microfilmed record containing information on other patients be left with a third party.

COMPETENCY CHECK: THREE

8. A patient with a large, overdue bill asks that his dental
records be transferred to another doctor. How does his
past-due account affect his right to have records transferred?

9. A medical assistant is served with a *subpoena duces
tecum*. With regard to the subpoenaed records, what is
her/his principal concern?

10. Before leaving subpoenaed records with anyone in a
courtroom, what should the custodian of the records
obtain?

11. A court may be willing to accept photocopied records
in lieu of the originals. However, what special precautions may have to be taken?

SUMMARY

Patient health care records have scientific, educational, financial, legal, and social purposes. However, despite the importance of the record and the fact that licensing regulations require hospitals to keep records, there is no specific regulation requiring that office medical records be kept. Clearly, however, it is in the best interests of all concerned to have such records.

Records are owned by the owner of the facility where treatment was provided (e.g., hospital, clinic, or doctor's office). At one time, they were not made available to patients. The law has now evolved to the point that a patient's right to the information in his/her medical record is as great as the hospital's or doctor's property right to the record. Consequently, patients must be given an opportunity to see the record and/or to obtain a copy of it.

Although there is agreement about providing the patient with information from his/her record, there are differing opinions about the form it should take. Some believe that a complete and unexpurgated copy of the record should be issued routinely and automatically to the patient. Others believe that dual records should be kept: a general excerpted record for the patient, and an active working record (with sensitive material, tentative hypotheses, etc.) for the doctor and other professionals involved in caring for the patient.

Laws regarding retention of patient records vary from state to state. It is generally agreed that, for the protection of the doctor, all patient records should be kept at least until all germane statutes of limitations have expired. Because statutes of limitations are extended for so many different reasons, however, it is preferable to keep records indefinitely.

The patient has the sole authority to release information from his/her record unless a legal disclosure is required. It should be noted, however, that when the record is subpoenaed, all legal and other necessary steps should be taken to protect the record.

When you have finished reading this chapter, complete the corresponding chapter in your workbook and then go to Chapter Eleven.

REFERENCES

1. Hirsh HL. Will your medical records get you into trouble? *Legal Aspects of Medical Practice.* September 1978;6:46.
2. Shenkin BN, Warner DC. Giving the patient his medical record. N Engl J Med. 1973;289:688.
3. Tucker G. Patient access to medical records. *Legal Aspects of Medical Practice.* August 1979;7:19-20.
4. Chapman S. How long should you keep your patient's medical records? *Legal Aspects of Medical Practice.* August 1979;7:19-20.
5. Preiser SE. The high cost of tampering with medical records. *Medical Economics.* April 20, 1992;69:195.
6. Ibid., 90.

11

Employment Safety and Rights Law

Many laws regulate the rights and responsibilities of employers, supervisors, and employees. Most of these regulations have become law within the past two decades.

At the present time, the relationship between employee and employer (as well as employee and supervisor) is more strictly circumscribed than ever before. Failure to comply with federal and state regulations can result in lawsuits as well as fines or other penalties.

OBJECTIVES:

After studying this chapter, you should be able to:

1. Describe the primary purposes of the workers compensation and OSHA laws.
2. Explain the responsibilities of both employer and employee under OSHA regulations.
3. List and explain the basic rules governing employer and employee rights and responsibilities in the following:

    a. Fair Labor Standards Act
    b. Civil Rights Act, Title VII
    c. Age Discrimination in Employment Act
    d. Americans with Disabilities Act
    e. Family and Medical Leave Act
    f. Immigration Reform

4. Outline a procedure, in compliance with Title VII, to prevent sexual harassment in the workplace.

As you read this chapter, remember that health care providers must comply with both federal and state laws. Individual state laws may set different and higher standards.

OCCUPATIONAL HEALTH AND SAFETY

Workers Compensation

The earliest employment legislation was concerned with workers injured on the job. The purpose of the legislation was: to provide, without regard to fault, medical care and compensation for the injured employee and his/her dependents; to provide rehabilitation, if necessary; to encourage employer interest in safety; and to promote safety in the workplace. Workers compensation insurance is mandated by federal and state law.

Occupational Safety and Health Act

The high number of work days lost due to job-related injuries prompted the passage of the federal Occupational Safety and Health Act (OSHA) of 1970, which applies to essentially all employers in the country. It was passed in an attempt to ensure that employees are provided with a workplace that is free from recognized hazards that cause serious injury or death. OSHA regulations cover the physical workplace, materials, machinery, and equipment, as well as first aid, protective clothing, and reporting requirements.

Employers must comply with all applicable OSHA standards, inform employees of OSHA requirements, keep specific records, compile and post an annual summary of work-related injuries and illnesses, provide safety training, require employees to wear safety equipment, and discipline employees for violations of safety rules. Employees must comply with OSHA standards, follow employer safety and health rules, use protective equipment and clothing when necessary, and report hazardous conditions. Employers may not discharge or discriminate against an employee for filing a complaint or testifying against an employer regarding OSHA violations.

OSHA inspectors may conduct inspections, issue citations for violations, and recommend penalties. Inspections are conducted in cases of imminent danger; catastrophic accidents resulting in the death or hospitalization of five or more employees; valid employee complaints; high-hazard occupations and industries; and follow up of previously investigated cases.

Right-to-know regulations give the health care employee and others the right to information about toxic hazards and the protective equipment to use when handling such materials. Toxic and poisonous chemicals, corrosive irritants, flammable materials, and carcinogens must have appropriate labels. Material safety data sheets (MSDS) for these products must be made available to employees. The MSDS lists each ingredient in the product. MSDS lists can be obtained from the manufacturers or prepared on site. In the case of a spill, the MSDS must be consulted to determine any hazards involved or necessary precautions that must be taken. Each incident requires documentation. The Standard for Occupational Exposures to Hazardous Chemicals in Laboratories further clarifies the handling of hazardous chemicals in medical laboratories.

COMPETENCY CHECK: ONE

1. Briefly explain the purposes of workers compensation legislation.

2. Why was the Occupational Safety and Health Act of 1970 enacted?

3. Do employees have any responsibilities under OSHA? Explain.

4. Why are right-to-know regulations important to health care providers? What is an MSDS?

Bloodborne Pathogens

Bloodborne pathogens, such as HIV and hepatitis B, are of particular concern to health care providers. Bloodborne pathogen standards pertain to blood and body fluids; the regulations cover both administrative and clinical aspects of practice. Body fluids include semen, blood, amniotic fluids, vaginal secretions, synovial fluid, pleural fluid, pericardial fluid, cerebrospinal fluid, and saliva.

OSHA's rules governing all freestanding health care providers affect more than 122,000 facilities nationwide. According to regulations, health care facilities must have:

1. A list of all employees who might be exposed to bloodborne diseases on either a regular or occasional basis.
2. A written exposure control plan.
3. One employee in charge of OSHA compliance.
4. Availability of protective equipment and clothing.
5. An employee training program in writing, and records of sessions and participants.
6. Warning labels and signs denoting biohazards.
7. Written guidelines for identifying, containing, and disposing of medical waste in accordance with state and local laws; the method for housecleaning and decontamination, including laundry.
8. Written guidelines for procedures to follow if an employee is exposed to blood or other potentially infectious materials, as well as a policy for reporting incidents of exposure and maintaining records.
9. Postexposure evaluation procedures.

Employers must also offer hepatitis B vaccine free of charge to every employee who can be reasonably anticipated to have contact with blood or other potentially infectious materials.

Medical Waste

Fear of AIDS and media coverage concerning the appearance of hazardous medical materials—such as syringes, needles, and scalpels—washing up on beaches has prompted legislative attention to the disposal of infectious and hazardous medical waste. Recent laws require that medical waste be handled with special care. Medical waste includes bandages; body specimens; diapers; disposable needles, syringes, scalpels, and other instruments; dressings; laboratory cultures; and radioactive materials.

The new legislation requires that medical waste be separated from other trash. Infectious wastes may be incinerated by the facility or placed in special puncture-resistant or lead-lined containers and removed by a medical waste disposal company. Waste must be tracked from the health care facility to the final incinerator or landfill. This tracking is accomplished through a system of identification labels, tracking forms, and logs.

Some states have passed laws that are stricter than the federal laws; consequently, it is important to be knowledgeable about the medical waste disposal laws for your state.

COMPETENCY CHECK: TWO

5. What are the nine requirements that medical offices must comply with under the bloodborne pathogen standards regulations?

6. Identify the nine body fluids covered in the regulations.

7. True or false: Employers must provide hepatitis B vaccine free of charge to certain employees.

8. True or false: Infectious medical waste must be put in plastic garbage bags before being placed in the garbage can.

FAIR LABOR PRACTICES

Fair Labor Standards Act of 1939

Both state and federal laws regulate wages, hours, and conditions of work. The Fair Labor Standards Act regulates the federal minimum wage, overtime compensation, equal pay requirements, child labor, and requirements for record keeping.

Minimum wages and overtime pay apply to all employees except employees such as executives, administrative personnel, professional employees, outside salespeople, agricultural workers, and state employees. These categories of employees are exempt from the federal overtime standards. All other employees are subject to the overtime standards, and are considered nonexempt.

For nonexempt employees, overtime is considered work exceeding 40 hours per week; time off may not be given in lieu of overtime pay.

If a receptionist spends his/her lunch period making the daily bank deposit or stays late to file x-rays, he/she is entitled to overtime pay if the work was permitted by the employer, even if it was not required by the employer.

An employer may dock a nonexempt employee for tardiness, but several rules must be considered. The policy must be known to employees beforehand, and must be applied fairly and without discrimination. The deduction must be made at the regular hourly rate of pay.

For example, if a pharmacy employed two pharmacy technicians on the day shift—one a young female who liked to go out at night and one a single mother who had three children—and both were frequently late for work, the employer could not dock the pay of the partying female, but ignore docking the pay of the single parent.

Social Security Act of 1935 and the Employee Retirement Income Security Act (ERISA) of 1974

The Social Security Act provides retirement benefits, disability benefits, dependent benefits, survivor benefits, and Medicare, while the Employee Retirement Income Security Act (ERISA) regulates and protects pensions.

COMPETENCY CHECK: THREE

9. True or False: The Fair Labor Standards Act established the federal minimum wage as well as rules for overtime compensation, equal pay, child labor, and record keeping requirements.

10. True or False: Overtime is considered work exceeding 50 hours per week.

11. If a file clerk comes in early to help catch up on work, is the employer required to pay overtime even if the employer did not ask the clerk to work extra hours?

12. What is provided by the Social Security Act?

Civil Rights Act of 1964 (1991)

One of the primary laws governing the relationships among employers, supervisors, and employees is Title VII of the Civil Rights Act of 1964, which makes discrimination in the workplace illegal. Title VII applies to employers that have fifteen employees or more for at least twenty weeks during the year; employment agencies; and local, state, and federal employers. The Equal Employment Opportunity Commission (EEOC) is the enforcing agency.

Title VII covers both discriminatory treatment and discriminatory impact. A job requirement may inadvertently be discriminatory if it is not really necessary for the job. If, for example, a height requirement is placed on the position of a physical therapist, the requirement could have a discriminatory impact on female physical therapists, since the average height of women is less than the average height of men. If a certain height is not really necessary for effective job performance, such a requirement could be discriminatory; if such a requirement is essential for performance of the job, then it would probably not be discriminatory.

Employers may not refuse to hire; limit, segregate, or classify; discharge; or otherwise discriminate against an individual with respect to compensation, conditions, or privileges of employment because of race, color, sex, religion, or national origin.

In addition to federal law, most of the states have enacted antidiscrimination statutes. Many state laws are more far-reaching than the federal statutes. Some state and local statutes prohibit discrimination on the basis of sexual orientation, personal appearance, mental health, mental retardation, marital status, parenthood, and political affiliation.

Care must be taken in hiring practices. For example, the following questions may not be asked on an application or in an interview:

1. **How old are you? What is your date of birth?** It is also unacceptable to require a photograph prior to hiring an applicant.

2. **Are you single or married?** Questions related to sex, children, birth control, child care, and family plans are illegal.
3. **Where were you born?** Questions regarding the birthplace of parents or spouse are also illegal. Any inquiry into the ancestry, national origin, or nationality of an applicant or the applicant's family is against the law. While information regarding the languages that an applicant can speak or write is acceptable, it is not legal to inquire about how the applicant learned the additional languages or which language is the first or primary language.
4. **What is your religious affiliation?**
5. **What is your maiden name?** Questions about an original name, if the name has been changed by court order or otherwise, are illegal. It *is* appropriate to inquire about reference material (e.g., educational, employment, and personal) that is under a different name.
6. **What is your height and weight?** Questions relating to an applicant's physical, medical, and mental status including height and weight are not allowed unless they directly relate to job requirements.
7. **Have you ever been arrested?** It is acceptable, however, to ask if an applicant has ever been convicted of a crime, and where, when, and what crime. A prospective employer may also ask if the applicant has any felony charges pending.
8. **In which country do you possess citizenship?** It is legal to ask if an applicant is a citizen of the United States, if the applicant has a legal right to reside in the U.S., and if the applicant intends to become a citizen and remain in the U.S. permanently.

Sexual Harassment

Sexual harassment has always been a common problem in the workplace. It has typically been directed toward women since they have been in lower positions and could not afford to lose their jobs. At the present time, however, with more women in supervisory positions, men are experiencing harassment more often than was formerly the case. Numerous court decisions in the last two decades have confirmed that this form of harassment is a cause for both criminal prosecution and civil litigation.

Sexual discrimination is illegal under Title VII of the Civil Rights Act; sexual harassment is considered to be a form of sex discrimination. In the seventies, the Equal Employment Opportunity Commission defined sexual harassment as unwelcome sexual advances or requests for sexual favors. In the eighties, the EEOC broadened the definition of sexual harassment to include other verbal or physical conduct of a sexual nature when: (1) submission to such conduct is made either explicitly or implicitly a term or condition of an individual's employment; (2) submission to or rejection of such conduct by an individual is used as a basis for employment decisions affecting such individual; or (3) such conduct has the purpose or effect of unreasonably interfering with an individual's work performance, or creating an intimidating, hostile, or offensive working environment.

The most common situation has been the demand by an employer or supervisor for sexual favors in exchange for job promotion or retention. This type of harassment is called *quid pro quo,* which means "this for that" in Latin. Another type of sexual harassment is the creation of an environment that is intimidating, hostile, or offensive which interferes with the individual's ability to perform creatively or effectively. This situation is most often associated with sexually explicit or gender-demeaning jokes, comments, or actions.

For example: In a facility that employed three male and one female x-ray technicians, the males frequently joked about PMS, the inferiority of females, and the proper role of the female being having babies and cleaning house. The supervising male technician referred to the female technician as "his girl," ignored suggestions made by the female but applauded similar suggestions when made by one of the males, and jokingly stated that the female technician was good enough for routine procedures, but he always assigned one of the others to "do the man's job" (e.g., IVPs and cholangiography). In this situation, the violation of the law would be characterized as "hostile environment" sexual harassment, not "quid pro quo" harassment.

Under the doctrine of *respondeat superior*, employers may be found liable even if the offense was caused by an employee. The employer is usually held liable if the harassment was caused by a supervisor. The harasser, as well as any management representative who knew or should have known about the harassment and condoned or ratified it, can be held personally liable for damages.

Not only is a program to purge sexual harassment from the workplace required by law, it is also the most practical way to avoid or limit damages if harassment should occur. Employers should implement a plan such as the following:

- Prepare a written policy stating that sexual harassment will not be tolerated.
- Offer education for employees with examples of sexual and gender harassment as well as gender discrimination.
- Develop a procedure for reporting incidents that ensures confidentiality.
- Provide prompt, thorough, and objective investigation of the situation. Interview anyone with information about the incident. Make a determination and convey the results to the complainant, the alleged harasser, and—as appropriate—all others directly concerned. Take appropriate action against the harasser. Take steps to prevent any further harassment. Immediately take appropriate action to remedy the complainant's loss, if any.

COMPETENCY CHECK: FOUR

13. **Some of the states have extended the prohibition against discrimination in employment to include which other groups?**

14. **Explain the meaning of sexual harassment according to Title VII.**

15. **True or False: An employer can be held responsible for the actions of an employee in a case of harassment.**

Age Discrimination in Employment Act (ADEA) of 1967 (1974)

The Age Discrimination in Employment Act of 1967 makes it illegal for employers with twenty or more employees to discriminate against workers on the basis of age. The protected age range is forty through sixty-five. Individual state laws may have different protected age ranges and less strict jurisdictional thresholds.

Americans with Disabilities Act (ADA) (1990)

The Americans with Disabilities Act (ADA) applies to employers with fifteen or more employees, including private employers, state and local governments, employment agencies, and labor unions. The ADA prohibits discrimination in all employment practices, including job application procedures, hiring, firing, advancement, compensation, training, and other terms, conditions, and privileges of employment. The act applies to recruitment, advertising, tenure, layoff, leave, fringe benefits, and all other related activities.

This statute applies to individuals with substantial (as distinct from minor) impairments. These must be impairments that limit major life activities. The law does not apply to individuals with minor nonchronic conditions of short duration, such as a broken arm or leg. The statute also protects persons with a history of cancer in remission, or a person with a history of mental illness, or a person with AIDS or who is HIV positive.

According to the ADA, a receptionist could not be fired following an auto accident that caused severe facial scarring just because the dentist-employer feared the "negative reactions" of others. An EKG technician, for example, with a positive HIV could not be fired because the physician-employers were afraid that patients would change health care providers out of fear of AIDS exposure.

No employer is required to hire a disabled applicant if the reason for not hiring the individual is unrelated to his/her disability and is pertinent to the position for which the individual is applying. If a medical transcriptionist with a disability types seventy words per minute accurately, but another applicant types ninety words per minute accurately, the employer may hire the applicant who types faster.

An employer can dismiss a disabled employee whose behavior is disruptive or whose performance is unacceptable. A bookkeeper with a history of alcoholism who is continually making errors can be fired if the termination is based on unsatisfactory performance, and warnings about the possible consequences of substandard work have been given and not heeded.

An employer must assure that a qualified individual with a disability has the same rights and privileges in employment as nondisabled applicants/employees. Reasonable accommodations must be made for the disabled employee. The employer is not required to make an accommodation if it would impose an "undue hardship," which is defined as "an action with significant difficulty or expense."

For example, if the building operations department of a large hospital was hiring a new engineer, and one of the routine duties involved working in the heating and ventilation duct system which measured 36 inches wide and 48 inches high, the employer would not be required to hire an applicant weighing 325 pounds. The applicant would be unable to fit into the duct system and replacing the system would be excessively expensive, if not impossible.

The following are examples of basic accommodations:

- Extra-wide parking spots as close as possible to the entrance reserved for the disabled.
- Gently inclined ramps or elevators.
- Easily opening doors, usually electric.
- Unobstructed hallways (pathways) with at least 36 inches of clearance.

- Bathroom handrails and facilities designed for the disabled.
- Accessible lounge, lunchroom, or cafeteria.
- Reception counters and other work areas that are low enough for a person in a wheelchair (maximum height of 34 inches).

While these are some examples of accommodations, it is possible that an employee with a back disability might simply require an ergonomically designed chair or a work area that is higher than the usual counter height in order to eliminate bending. For example, a receptionist with a neck disability might require a headset for the telephone. An employee who is confined to a wheelchair may need an office that opens directly into a main hall or outside area.

> Experts who have studied the ADA don't expect government regulators and judges to be unreasonable. "Fully accessible," for example, doesn't necessarily apply to every part of the building. And the law doesn't insist on immediate compliance if that would impose financial hardship. In many cases, inexpensive or temporary fixes may be adequate to demonstrate efforts to comply. For instance, instead of a costly automatic door and a concrete ramp, you might get by with a doorbell and a wood ramp. You might install a wheelchair lift for $10,000 instead of spending $40,000 or more for a new elevator.[1]

An employer may not make a preemployment inquiry on an application form or in an interview as to whether, or to what extent, an individual is disabled. The employer may ask a job applicant whether he/she can perform particular job functions. If the applicant has a disability known to the employer, the employer may ask how he/she can perform job functions that the employer considers difficult or impossible to perform because of the disability, and whether an accommodation would be needed. A job offer may be conditioned on the results of a medical examination, provided that the exam is required for all entering employees in the same job category with or without disability, and that information obtained is handled according to confidentiality requirements specified in the act.

The ADA does take safety issues into consideration. The law expressly permits employers to establish qualification standards that will exclude individuals who pose a direct threat (i.e., a significant risk to the health and safety of others) if that risk cannot be lowered to an acceptable level by reasonable accommodations.

Individuals who are currently engaged in the illegal use of drugs are specifically excluded from the definition of a "qualified individual with a disability" protected by the ADA when actions are taken because of their drug use.

The employment provisions of the ADA are enforced under the same policies now applicable to race, sex, national origin, and religious discrimination under Title VII. Complaints may be filed with the EEOC or a designated state human rights agency. Remedies will include hiring, reinstatement, back pay, and court orders to stop discrimination. Employers who have been found guilty of intentional discrimination can be required to pay compensatory damages, attorneys' fees, and possibly punitive damages if they acted with reckless indifference to the employee's rights, or with malice.

COMPETENCY CHECK: FIVE

16. True or False: The Americans with Disabilities Act applies to persons with any impairment.

17. True or False: No employer is required to hire a disabled applicant if the reason for the hiring is unrelated to the disability and is pertinent to the employment.

18. True or False: Reasonable accommodations must be made for the disabled employee.

19. True or False: If an employer is found guilty of malice and discrimination against a disabled worker, the court may allow punitive damages as well as compensatory damages and attorneys' fees.

Family and Medical Leave Act of 1993

Federal and state laws require employers covered by the Family and Medical Leave Act of 1993 to provide up to twelve weeks per year of unpaid, job-protected leave to eligible employees for certain family and medical reasons. Employees are eligible if they have worked for a covered employer for at least one year, and for 1,250 hours over the previous twelve months.

Unpaid leave must be granted for the following reasons:

- to enable an employee to care for his/her child after birth, adoption, or foster care placement.
- to enable an employee to care for a spouse, child, or parent who has a serious health condition.
- for a serious health condition that makes the employee unable to perform his/her job.

Certain types of paid leave may be substituted for unpaid leave if agreed to by both the employee and employer. The employee ordinarily must provide thirty days advance notice when the leave is foreseeable. An employer may require medical certification to support a request for leave because of a serious health condition. The employer may also require second or third medical opinions (at the employer's expense) and a fitness for duty report to return to work.

For the duration of the leave, the employer must maintain the employee's coverage under any group health plan.

Upon return from the leave, most employees must be restored to their original or equivalent positions with equivalent pay, benefits, and other employment terms. The use of the leave cannot result in the loss of any employment benefit that accrued prior to the start of the employee's leave.

It is unlawful for the employer to interfere with, restrain, or deny the exercise of any right provided under the law; or to discharge or discriminate against any person for opposing any practice made unlawful by the law; or for being involved in any proceedings under or relating to the law. The U.S. Department of Labor is authorized to investigate and resolve complaints of violations brought under the federal law. An eligible employee may also bring a civil action against an employer for violations.

Immigration Reform (1986)

The Immigration Reform and Control Act was the first major revision of immigration policy in the United States in decades. The basic purposes of the act were to:

- preserve jobs for those who are legally entitled to them: American citizens and aliens who are authorized to work in this country.
- prohibit employers with four or more employees from discriminating against any authorized individual in hiring, discharging, or recruiting because of national origin or citizenship status.

There are severe penalties for employers found to be noncompliant, including fines and imprisonment. The Handbook for Employers on Instructions for Completing Federal Form I-9 from the U.S. Government Printing Office contains information, instructions, reproductions of Form I-9, and documents that establish identity and employment eligibility.

Documents that can be used to establish both identity and employment eligibility include a United States passport; certificate of U.S. citizenship; certificate of naturalization; unexpired employment authorization document issued by the Immigration and Naturalization Service (INS) containing a photograph; alien registration receipt card with photo; unexpired temporary resident card; unexpired employment authorization card; unexpired reentry permit; unexpired refugee travel document; and unexpired employment foreign passport with I-551 stamp or INS form I-94 indicating unexpired employment authorization.

COMPETENCY CHECK: SIX

20. The Family and Medical Leave Act allows unpaid leave for what reasons?

21. How many weeks per year of unpaid leave is allowed for each employee?

22. Explain the employer's obligation regarding the employee's position, pay, and benefits under this act.

SUMMARY

In the past, employers had a great deal of control over hiring and firing, conditions of employment, and working environment.

Certain laws seek to protect the health, welfare, and safety of employees. Workers compensation laws provide compensation to the employee and dependents for work-related illness and injury, provide rehabilitation, and encourage safety in the workplace. The occupational safety and health laws require employers and employees to strive for greater safety. Right-to-know regulations give employees the right to be informed about what toxic and hazardous substances are being used in the workplace and what necessary safety precautions must be taken.

Bloodborne pathogen standards pertain to health care providers who are exposed to blood and body fluids that could be contaminated by HIV, hepatitis B, or other pathogens.

The Social Security Act (SSA) and the Employee Retirement Income Security Act (ERISA) provide retirement benefits and regulate and protect private pension plans. Labor practices have been affected by numerous pieces of legislation. The Fair Labor Standards Act (FLSA) addresses the issues of minimum wage, overtime compensation, equal pay requirements, child labor, and basic issues of discrimination. Title VII of the Civil Rights Act of 1964 is one of the primary laws governing relations among employers, supervisors, and employees. Title VII prohibits discrimination in labor practices and includes prohibitions against sexual harassment. The Age Discrimination in Employment Act (ADEA) and the Americans with Disabilities Act (ADA) have all protected the rights of specific groups to enter or remain in the work force.

The Immigration Reform and Control Act of 1986 prohibits the employment of illegal aliens. It was intended to protect citizens and legal aliens from loss of employment, and also to protect legal aliens from discrimination based on national origin or citizenship.

The recent legislation covered in this chapter, as well as other federal and state legislation, has had a great impact on employees' sense of security. It has had an equally great impact on the ability of employers to deal with uncooperative or unproductive employees and operate a business profitably. It is necessary to be aware of current issues and laws at the federal, state, and local levels.

When you have finished reading this chapter, complete the corresponding chapter in your workbook and then go to the Chapter Twelve.

REFERENCES

1. Rice B. Does your office meet the new standards for the disabled? *Medical Economics.* April 20, 1992;69:195.

12

Consumer Protection Laws

Since credit arrangements and collection procedures are important parts of the business aspects of health care, there are a number of consumer protection laws that are pertinent to health care law and ethics. It is essential that those who deal with these aspects of practice be careful to comply with federal, state, and local statutes.

OBJECTIVES

After studying this chapter, you will be able to:

1. Explain the concept of professional courtesy.
2. Outline the rule of confidentiality as it applies to financial information.
3. Explain the Equal Credit Opportunity Act of 1975.
4. Explain the purpose of the Fair Credit Reporting Act of 1971.
5. Identify the charges that the American Medical Association consider unethical.
6. Identify the significance of the statute of frauds in collections.
7. Explain the terms of Regulation Z of the Consumer Protection Act of 1969 (Truth in Lending.)
8. Identify the major provisions of the Fair Debt Collections Practices Act of 1978.
9. Explain the significance of each of the following in relation to the collection of debts:

   A. Statutes of limitations
   B. Small claims court
   C. Garnishment
   D. Liens in personal injury cases
   E. Bankruptcy (Revised Bankruptcy Act of 1979)
   F. Claims against estates

FINANCIAL PHILOSOPHY AND PROCEDURE

In all types of practices, it is necessary to develop a credit and collections policy. All federal and state legislation must be considered while establishing policies for granting credit, collecting fees, credit card billing, health insurance reimbursement, billing, and collection follow-up procedures. It is essential to discuss the policy and procedures with all office staff. Such policies and procedures should be followed by all employees and should be applied equally to all patients.

PROFESSIONAL COURTESY

Professional courtesy is actually a discount or waiver of fees. Traditionally, physicians have treated other physicians and their family members without charging a fee. This courtesy is commonly extended to members of the clergy and their family members, and to health care professionals who are employed in the doctor's office, offices of associates, or the hospital.

The entire fee can be waived or a percentage of the fee can be discounted. If a patient receiving professional courtesy insists upon paying, the payment should be accepted. If a physician's family member requests a statement for the services, the notation "by request" or "at patient's request" should appear on the statement.

CONFIDENTIALITY

The basic rule of confidentiality of information applies to the financial records of a patient just as it does to the medical records of a patient. Disclosure of a patient's financial information should only be made with the written authorization of the patient or as required by law. Federal and state laws have been enacted to protect the rights of consumers. A facility policy should be established according to these regulations.

1. True or false: Professional courtesy is commonly extended to members of the clergy.

2. True or false: Confidentiality does not apply to the financial information regarding a patient.

EQUAL CREDIT OPPORTUNITY ACT OF 1975

The Equal Credit Opportunity Act of 1975 prohibits discrimination in the granting of credit. The law prohibits discrimination based on race, color, national origin, age, sex, marital status or religion; in addition, persons who receive public assistance or those who have exercised their rights under consumer credit laws cannot be discriminated against.

FAIR CREDIT REPORTING ACT OF 1971

The purpose of the Fair Credit Reporting Act is to allow a person to see and correct his/her credit report. If credit is denied to a patient based on a negative credit report from a credit reporting agency, the patient must be notified. It is not necessary to inform the patient about the specifics, but failure to notify the patient and supply the name and address of the reporting agency can result in legal action.

CHARGES TO BE AVOIDED

The Council on Ethical and Judicial Affairs of the American Medical Association is responsible for interpreting the *AMA Principles of Medical Ethics*. The opinions or interpretations are periodically published as a guide for physicians.

The following fees are considered ethical, if the patient is notified in advance: fees for multiple or complex insurance forms (but not the first form); interest or finance charges; and fees for missed appointments that have not been canceled within a specific time. A patient information brochure is the best way to inform patients about facility/practice policies, but notations may be made on statements, or a notice may be posted in the reception area.

STATUTE OF FRAUDS

All states have laws, known as the statute of frauds, that specify which contracts must be written in order to be enforceable. A contract must be in writing if a third party agrees to be responsible for the debts of another and if the contract will extend beyond one year. (See Chapter Three.)

TRUTH IN LENDING ACT (REGULATION Z)

Sometimes patients require an extended period of time to pay dental and medical debts. Bills for surgery, orthodontia, fertility procedures, hospitalization, physical therapy, and obstetrics are examples of installment payment situations.

The Truth in Lending Act (also known as Regulation Z of the Consumer Protection Act of 1969) requires that there be a written agreement for payment of fees if: (1) there is a bilateral agreement; and (2) the fee is to be paid in more than four installments. It does not matter whether interest is charged; a truth in lending statement must be prepared. However, if the patient *unilaterally* decides to pay for services in more than four installments, the truth in lending statement is not required.

Although most health care providers do not charge interest on installment payments, it is legally and ethically acceptable to do so. The required elements of Regulation Z include the following:

1. total amount of the debt;
2. amount of the down payment;
3. date that each payment is due;
4. date that the final payment is due;
5. amount of each payment;
6. finance charges;
7. interest rate expressed as an annual percentage;
8. the patient and the physician or representative must sign the form; and
9. the patient and physician should each retain a copy of the completed form.

COMPETENCY CHECK: TWO

3. List four of the factors that cannot be used to decide whether to grant credit to a patient.

4. True or false: The Fair Credit Reporting Act of 1971 requires that a patient who is turned down for credit based on a negative credit report be informed of the specific information received.

5. List three charges that are considered acceptable by the AMA if the patient is informed in advance.

6. True or false: The statute of limitations identifies those contracts that must be in writing to be valid.

7. True or false: A truth in lending statement must be prepared only when interest is being charged.

8. State the two criteria that indicate the need for a truth in lending statement.

STATUTE OF LIMITATIONS

The statute of limitations indicates the length of time in which legal action can be initiated for various types of legal matters. There is a statute of limitations for breach of contract actions, which can include attempts to collect a debt. The time limit is not the same in each state, nor is it the same for different types of contracts.

FAIR DEBT COLLECTIONS PRACTICES ACT OF 1978

The Fair Debt Collections Practices Act of 1978 outlines collection practices for creditors. It prohibits and regulates many types of collection practices. One part of the act protects consumers against harassment resulting from a creditor making illegal or empty threats, practicing deceptive or unfair methods, or using abusive language. For example, if the collection manager of a podiatry office told a patient that his/her delinquent account would be sent to a collection agency unless payment was received within ten days, and the account was not referred to the collection agency at the end of that time, the patient could sue for harassment.

When pursuing collection of past-due accounts, it is important that there is no misrepresentation, harassment, or threats. Patients can be contacted during reasonable hours and cannot be contacted more frequently than once a week. In general, a patient's privacy must be protected. Violation of the FDCPA can result in suits based on invasion of privacy, defamation of character, and other tort grounds.

SMALL CLAIMS COURT

Small claims court can be useful in collecting overdue accounts. Each state—and sometimes a judicial district of a state—possesses a specific minimum and maximum dollar amount that can be taken to small claims court. The small claims court process then proceeds as follows: A claim is filed for a small fee, the defendant is served with a summons, and the plaintiff is notified when to appear. Then, each party brings evidence and witnesses to court, the judge questions each party, reviews the evidence, and makes a ruling. If the plaintiff wins a judgment, there is a legal right to garnish/attach wages, bank accounts, personal property, or real property.

Federal Wage Garnishment Law (1970)

Under the Federal Wage Garnishment Law, creditors are allowed to attach a debtor's wages and property. The amount of employee earnings that may be withheld for garnishment in any workweek or pay period is limited. The employee is protected from being fired if his/her pay is garnisheed for only one debt. There are some exceptions to the law. Additional information can be obtained from the United States Department of Labor.

COMPETENCY CHECK: THREE

9. True or false: The purpose of the Fair Debt Collections Practices Act is to prevent harassment by creditors.

10. State at least two collection practices that are illegal.

LIENS IN PERSONAL INJURY CASES

A lien is an encumbrance upon property to satisfy or protect a claim for payment of a debt. When services are being rendered to a patient who has obtained the services of an attorney, and a claim is made against another person for causing the patient's injury, a lien can be executed. The lien ensures that the doctor or facility is paid from any sums received by the patient from the adverse party. The lien is signed by the patient and the patient's attorney and kept by the provider of services.

BANKRUPTCY

Federal bankruptcy laws are designed to accomplish two main goals: (1) to provide relief and protection to debtors who have become insolvent (incapable of paying debts); and (2) to provide a fair method of distributing a debtor's assets among all creditors.

If a patient files under Chapter VII of the law, called straight bankruptcy, the assets are converted to funds by the trustee and distributed among the creditors. Creditors must not continue any collection procedures. This means that regular billing for services to that date must cease even if the patient is not currently a collection problem.

Under Chapter XIII of the law, called wage earner's bankruptcy, wage earners are provided with a means of paying off their debts free from the harassment of creditors.

The wage earner pays a specific amount to the trustee in bankruptcy; the trustee then distributes the money among the creditors.

During this three-year period, creditors cannot attach the debtor's wages or pursue any other collection procedures. When notified that a patient/debtor has filed a petition of bankruptcy, all collections efforts must cease and the creditor may file a claim with the bankruptcy court.

A creditor can be fined for contempt of court for failure to comply with the bankruptcy laws.

CLAIMS AGAINST ESTATES

Statements for bills owed by a deceased patient need to be sent, after a reasonable period of time, to the estate of the deceased patient, in care of the spouse or next of kin. The statement of account may not be sent to a relative unless there is a written agreement indicating that the relative is responsible for the debts of the deceased.

A request may be sent to the probate department of the superior court in the county in which the estate will be settled if the name of the responsible relative, the executor, or the administrator of the estate is unknown. There will be a specific time limit to file a claim against an estate. If the claim is denied, there are legal procedures provided to further pursue the claim. Time limits and procedures for collection of an account against an estate vary from state to state.

COMPETENCY CHECK: FOUR

11. Why would a doctor want to obtain a lien in the case of services rendered to a patient hurt in an auto accident?

12. What are the two basic purposes of federal bankruptcy laws?

SUMMARY

Careful management of the business side of health care, including a positive philosophy and well-defined credit and collection procedures, is vitally important. A number of laws govern the granting of credit and the collection of debts. Most of this legislation is designed to protect consumers from discrimination and harassment.

The Equal Credit Opportunity Act of 1975 prohibits discrimination in granting credit. The Fair Credit Reporting Act of 1971 protects the rights of consumers. The Fair Debt Collections Practices Act of 1978 protects debtors from harassment, threats, and abusive collection practices.

The Truth in Lending Act requires creditors to issue a truth in lending statement in certain circumstances.

The statute of limitations specifies the time allowed to initiate legal action, and the statute of frauds indicates which contracts must be in writing in order to be enforceable.

Creditors may elect to use small claims court to collect accounts when patients breach their contractual obligations to pay for services rendered. A lien or garnishment can assist in collections.

The federal bankruptcy laws are intended to give insolvent debtors relief from creditors while the debtor's assets are distributed among creditors.

There are some charges that are considered acceptable by the American Medical Association only if the patient is notified in advance.

When you have finished reading this chapter, complete the corresponding chapter in your workbook and then proceed to Chapter 13.

13

Litigation and Other Means of Preventing and Resolving Conflict

To acquaint you with the procedural rules governing civil lawsuits, this chapter will summarize the litigation process. Also, the most common causes of problems between health care providers and patients will be examined, and preventative measures discussed. Remember, it is easier to prevent professional liability claims than to defend them.

OBJECTIVES

After studying this chapter on litigation and other means of preventing and resolving conflict, you will be able to:

1. Explain the differences among the four phases of the litigation process: pleadings, pretrial discovery, trial, and appeals.
2. Explain complaint, answer, and reply.
3. Identify and explain the procedures for gathering information during the pretrial discovery phase.
4. Sequence the events that occur in a civil trial.
5. Discuss the guidelines for filing an appeal.
6. Review the causes of litigation (other than actual negligence) against health care providers.
7. Explain the concept of quality assurance/risk management in health care facilities.
8. Itemize six preventative guidelines for avoiding litigation and conflict between health care professionals and patients.

CAUSES OF CONFLICT

As discussed in Chapter One, there are many reasons for the increase in lawsuits against health care professionals.

The media has had a significant effect on the perceptions of the American public about health care and health care providers.

The underlying cause of many cases of litigation is the breakdown of the rapport between health care provider and patient. One of the most frequent complaints heard by medical society grievance committees is that the patient did not believe the health care professional gave sympathetic counsel in addition to professional care. The lack of a clear, complete explanation of the patient's health problem was another frequent complaint.

RESOLUTION OF CONFLICT

The Litigation Process

If a dispute between two individuals cannot be settled privately, the party who feels wronged (the plaintiff) may retain an attorney to seek a legal remedy. Often the attorney tries to settle the case out of court before instituting formal legal proceedings. If this effort fails, the attorney begins the usually lengthy and expensive litigation process on behalf of his/her client.

Pleadings Phase

The first phase of the suit is called the *pleadings* phase. The pleadings consist primarily of three legal documents designed to identify the controversial or disputed issues to be decided during trial. Only material relevant to issues described in the pleadings may be presented during trial. The pleadings usually consist of the *complaint*, the *answer*, and the *reply*.

The complaint. Through his/her attorney, the plaintiff files in court a written statement setting forth the basis of the claim against the defendant demanding a certain amount of monetary compensation for the alleged wrongdoing. (In some jurisdictions, the complaint is known as the petition or declaration.)

The complaint and a summons are then served on the defendant by a court representative. These comprise the defendant's official notice of the suit and require the defendant to appear in court at a certain time to defend himself/herself.

Not responding to a summons, which is known as defaulting, usually results in a judgment against the defendant. An example:

> A physician prescribed a drug that allegedly caused kidney failure in the patient. The patient sued the physician for negligence. The physician did not respond to the complaint/summons served on him, and the clerk entered a default decision against him. The physician was then ordered to appear in court and did so once, but failed to appear at a hearing.
>
> As a result, the court decided the suit in favor of the patient and awarded him $354,318.75 in damages. The physician appealed, but the appellate court upheld the verdict. The court commented that the physician was an intelligent, well-educated person who knew what was happening but failed to take appropriate action. (*Sawyer v Cox*, 244 S.E.2d 173, N.C. 1978)

Through his/her attorney, the defendant may file with the court a motion (called a demurrer) to have the case against him/her dismissed on the grounds that the plaintiff's complaint does not describe a legitimate legal claim. If the judge grants the defendant's motion, the case is dismissed; if the motion is denied, the next step in the pleadings phase occurs.

The answer. This is the defendant's written response to the allegations presented in the plaintiff's complaint. Affirmative defenses and counterclaims, if any, must be stated in the defendant's answer. In most jurisdictions, the law requires that the answer be filed with the court within 15-20 days.

The reply. In some jurisdictions, the plaintiff may file a response—the reply—to the defendant's answer. In other jurisdictions, it is assumed that the defendant's defense is denied.

Pretrial Discovery Phase

The next phase in the litigation process is called the pretrial discovery phase. The main purpose of this period is to permit the parties to uncover all relevant information before trial. Pretrial discovery helps to ensure that the dispute is settled fairly and on the issues, rather than on the ability of one litigant to surprise the other with concealed evidence.

During the pretrial discovery phase, each party has the right to obtain information through one or more of the following procedures:

1. **Interrogatories.** An interrogatory is a list of written questions prepared by one litigant and served on the other. The questions must be answered in writing and under oath.
2. **Depositions.** A deposition is a statement made under oath by a witness or potential witness in a question and answer form. The questions are posed by an attorney and the responses of the witness are recorded verbatim by a court reporter who transcribes the proceeding. Both sides may be present during the taking of a deposition and the witness may be cross-examined by opposing counsel. Depositions may be, and often are, introduced as evidence during trial.
3. **Court orders.** A court order is a direction or instruction by the court for one party to produce documents or other objects for inspection and duplication by the other party. A court may also order an injured party to submit to a physical and/or mental examination when the party's condition is in dispute. Depending on the circumstances, the examination may be performed by a court-appointed physician or a physician selected by either party.
4. **Requests for admissions.** Requests for admissions are written lists of assertions that one party asks the other to admit or deny. If the adverse party denies an assertion later proved true by the other party, the

adverse party may have to pay the costs involved in proving the assertion.

The following hypothetical case (summarized from a case cited in *Medical Malpractice*, 1974, Chapter Ten, 10-12, 29; copyright 1982 by Matthew Bender & Co.; used with permission) illustrates how an attorney may use the pretrial discovery period and its techniques to uncover relevant information. Although this case presents only the plaintiff's side, defense attorneys use the same procedures to uncover information substantiating their clients' positions. One tool used more frequently by defendants' attorneys than by plaintiffs' attorneys is the court order requiring the injured party (normally, the plaintiff) to submit to a physical or mental examination by an independent, court-appointed physician. The purpose of this examination is to obtain an impartial opinion on the extent of the injuries.

Background: Mr. Jones, a 58-year-old barber, complained to his family doctor that varicose veins in his legs were bothering him. His physician, Dr. A, recommended removal of the veins. He told Mr. Jones it would be a minor operation that would require hospitalization for a day or so. Mr. Jones consented. Dr. A performed the operation at the community hospital using a general anesthesia.

Upon awakening after surgery, the patient experienced more pain in his left leg than he had anticipated and noticed that surgery had not been performed on his right leg. Dr. A told him only that his hospital stay would be longer than expected and that surgery on his right leg should be postponed. During the next few days, the patient was examined several times by Dr. A and by two other physicians, Drs. B and C, none of whom explained to Mr. Jones' satisfaction why surgery on his right leg was postponed or why his hospital stay was extended.

A few days after the original operation, all three doctors advised Mr. Jones to have another operation on his left leg to remove a blood clot. He consented. The operation was performed by Dr. C, a cardiovascular surgeon, and eight days later the patient was discharged. Soon after arriving home, Mr. Jones and his wife noticed that his left leg was swollen and blue; the next day it had turned black. Dr. A told Mr. Jones to return immediately to the hospital. There, all three doctors recommended a below-knee-amputation of Mr. Jones' leg and Mr. Jones consented.

His recovery was thereafter uneventful, but Mr. Jones did not receive what he considered a satisfactory explanation of what went wrong. After the hospital refused to show him his records, he consulted an attorney. When the attorney was unable to obtain the records, Mr. Jones asked him to file suit against Dr. A. The attorney agreed, and within a few weeks Dr. A was served with a summons and copy of the plaintiff's complaint. *(In the case described here, the patient had to initiate the litigation process before being permitted to see his hospital records. In recent years, however, legislation has made it possible for patients to see their records before going to the expense and trouble of filing a lawsuit.)*

Pretrial discovery. Plaintiff's attorney decided to take Dr. A's deposition so that he could question Dr. A face-to-face and follow up his answers. The atmosphere during a deposition is informal (compared to trials) and the rules of admissibility and relevance enforced during a trial are not as strictly applied. Even so, each side knows that if it abuses its right and powers, thereby necessitating a court ruling on the procedure, the offending attorney or client may be personally assessed certain court costs.

Taking Dr. A's deposition proved to be informative for the attorney. First, he learned that general practitioners commonly performed varicose vein surgery in Dr. A's community. Secondly, he learned that Dr. A's only assistant was a scrub nurse assigned by the hospital. Thirdly, he learned that just as Dr. A was tying off what he thought was the saphenous vein in the patient's leg, Dr. B entered the operating room and "sort of took over the operation."

Dr. B, a general surgeon, told Dr. A that the femoral artery had been severed and that he, Dr. B, would try to repair it. After this effort was concluded, both physicians proceeded with the vein surgery on the left leg but postponed surgery on the right. Dr. A then said that a blood clot formed a few days later, necessitating a second operation by a vascular surgeon, Dr. C. When the clot recurred, gangrene set in and the leg had to be amputated.

Plaintiff's attorney then decided to take Dr. B's deposition. Since Dr. B was not, at that point, a litigant, a subpoena was served on him. The defendant, Dr. A, and his attorney were notified, so that they could attend the deposition.

Dr. B testified that he was in the hospital at the time of the surgery on Mr. Jones and that he was summoned to the operating site by the nurse in charge of the operating room. She said Dr. A appeared to be having some trouble. When Dr. B entered the room, he realized that Dr. A had divided the femoral artery into two ligatures, one of which had been tied by the scrub nurse and the other by Dr. A. He said that, with Dr. A's permission, he attempted to repair the artery. He stated he was a qualified general surgeon, but not a vascular surgeon. He further stated that Dr. A asked him to help proceed with the original surgery on the patient's left leg so that the patient would not suspect anything was wrong.

Because both Dr. B and Dr. A feared the possibility of a blood clot in the artery, they asked a vascular surgeon, Dr. C, to enter the case. When the clot did occur, Dr. C performed the second operation. Despite the use of anticoagulants, the clot recurred, gangrene developed, and the patient's leg had to be amputated.

The plaintiff's attorney hypothesized that the effectiveness of the anticoagulants was reduced because of the vein surgery and asked Dr. B for his opinion. Dr. B refused, on advice of defendant's attorney, on the basis that an expert witness is not required to respond to such questions from an adverse party. Thereafter, the deposition was concluded.

The attorney then decided to take Dr. C's deposition, but Dr. C had had a heart attack and had been advised by his attending physician to avoid stressful situations. The plaintiff's attorney decided, therefore, to use a procedure known as a "deposition on written questions." He prepared a list of questions and cross-questions and delivered them to a court officer who posed them to the witness. Through this procedure, the attorney was able to confirm testimony given by Drs. A and B and establish the extent of Dr. C's involvement.

After studying the information uncovered during the depositions, the attorney changed plaintiff's complaint to include Dr. B, the scrub nurse, and the hospital as codefendants. He then obtained a court order permitting him to inspect and copy the hospital records.

Next, the attorney served each physician-defendant with an interrogatory. Its purpose was to learn which medical texts each physician had in his medical library on the subjects of varicose veins and gangrene. (In most jurisdictions an attorney may cross-examine expert witnesses only on those medical texts the expert says he/she has used or depended upon.)

The hospital was asked to admit or deny:

- that the scrub nurse was regularly employed by the hospital.
- that the nurse was assigned as a scrub nurse, not a surgical assistant, to the operation performed on Mr. Jones.
- that the procedure of ligating a vein or artery is not one to be performed by a scrub nurse under hospital rules.

This "request for admissions" was the final discovery technique the plaintiff's attorney used to prepare for the trial.

After both sides have had a fair chance to obtain relevant information, the trial judge often calls a pretrial conference to try to settle the case before the expense of a trial, or to simplify and clarify the relevant issues. This conference is attended by the judge and attorneys for both sides; the parties may attend if they wish. If the dispute is not settled, the trial phase of the litigation process begins.

Trial Phase

The purpose of the trial is to hear the case in a neutral environment and to achieve a just settlement to the dispute. During the trial, the judge acts as a referee, so to speak, to ensure that both sides proceed in a fair, legally-required manner. At any time in the litigation process, the parties are free to settle the matter among themselves and are often encouraged to do so. The most important steps in a trial are briefly described here and usually occur in the same order as presented.

1. The first step is to select a jury, unless the parties agree to a "bench trial." In a bench trial, the judge hears the case, decides the facts, and renders the verdict.

    Selecting a jury is an art unto itself. Each side attempts to select jurors sympathetic to its position. Experienced trial lawyers have developed their own methods of selecting jurors.

    The task of the jury is to hear and decide the facts of the case. The presiding judge decides all issues of law and explains them to the jury.
2. After the jury is selected, each side presents an opening statement of what it expects to prove.
3. The plaintiff then presents his/her evidence. Witnesses are called. They are first questioned under direct examination by plaintiff's attorney. The

defendant's attorney may cross-examine each witness; often the goal of cross-examination is to discredit or confuse the witness.

4. After plaintiff has presented his/her evidence, the defendant begins his/her case. His/her first action may be to move for a directed verdict for himself/herself if he/she believes the plaintiff has not substantiated the charges against the defendant. If the judge agrees, he/she directs the jury to grant the motion and dismiss the case. If the judge denies the motion, the defense presents its evidence and case. Witnesses are called and examined. The plaintiff is given an opportunity to cross-examine defense witnesses. After its evidence has been presented, the defense "rests."

5. The plaintiff then may produce evidence to rebut the defendant's evidence.

6. The defendant may again move for a directed verdict on his/her behalf. If the motion is granted, the case is dismissed; if denied, each side presents closing arguments.

7. After closing arguments, the judge instructs the jury on the law and on how to determine appropriate money damages, if applicable. This step is sometimes called the judge's charge or instructions to the jury. The judge says that if the jury finds that certain facts were established, the jury must find for the plaintiff. If the jury believes the plaintiff did not prove certain facts or that an affirmative defense was proved by the defendant, the jury must find for the defendant. Among the judge's instructions will be the reminder that in civil suits the plaintiff must prove his/her case by a *preponderance of evidence*. In other words, plaintiff's evidence must be greater than defendant's. In criminal cases the evidence must show the defendant *guilty beyond a reasonable doubt*.

8. The jury is then sequestered to discuss the issues and reach a verdict. If the jury is unable to reach a

decision, it is considered a "hung jury," and a new trial will be ordered by the court. If the jury reaches a verdict, it reports it to the judge; the judge then renders the judgment according to the jury's verdict.

Appeals Phase

After a verdict has been declared, the losing side may appeal the decision to a higher court. However, one does not have an automatic right to a case review by an appellate court. Appellate court reviews are granted only when the evidence suggests the strong possibility of error, injustice, or impropriety during the trial court proceedings. The appeal must be based on an issue of law, rather than on the jury's decision concerning a fact.

If an appellate court agrees to hear the case, written statements by both sides are presented and oral arguments heard. Appeals courts consist of three, five, seven, or nine judges, and decisions are made by majority vote. Appellate courts have the power to affirm, modify, set aside, or reverse trial court decisions. They also have the power to order a new trial.

A judgment cannot be considered final until all options for appeal have been exercised.

COMPETENCY CHECK: ONE

1. **List and briefly describe the four basic phases of the litigation process.**

2. **List the following in the order each would normally occur: answer; closing statements; opening statements; complaint; depositions; judgment; defendant's evidence; jury selection; appeal; plaintiff's evidence; verdict.**

Alternatives for Resolving Disputes

To reduce the load on the overburdened judicial system, solutions for ways to resolve disputes outside the courtroom have been sought. The two most common alternatives are joint screening panels and arbitration panels, both of which can be valuable and workable alternatives, in some instances, to the litigation process.

Joint screening panels. These are usually composed of attorneys and physicians and, in some cases, a representative of the public. The panel reviews a patient's claim and advises whether a suit should be pursued or dropped. If the panel believes the plaintiff's claim has merit, it may agree to help the plaintiff obtain expert medical testimony; if it believes the plaintiff's complaint is without merit, it expects the matter to be dropped. In most jurisdictions, the decision of the screening panel is not binding on either party. Normally, screening panels neither make a judgment nor give advice regarding monetary compensation. The composition and jurisdiction of screening panels, their procedures and requirements for hearing cases, and the impact of their decisions vary from state to state. Their common goals, however, are to eliminate claims that have no merit and to help plaintiffs with legitimate claims to obtain expert witnesses.

Joint screening panels should not be confused with the physician review panels established by many medical societies. Physician review panels are composed solely of physicians from a particular medical society. When a member of that society is notified that he/she is being sued, he/she informs the panel, which reviews the case and advises the physician and his/her insurance carrier on whether to settle the claim or to prepare a defense.

Arbitration. Arbitration is another way of settling disputes out of court. Although similar to screening panels in that a panel of impartial people is convened to hear a case, arbitration boards have much broader scope and authority. The arbitration process is intended to be a complete substitute for the litigation process. When the two parties voluntarily agree to submit a dispute to arbitration, or when arbitration is required by state law, the decision of the panel is considered final, binding, and enforceable by the courts. Several states require that disputes involving a relatively small amount of money (less than $10,000) be subject to arbitration. However, the right of the loser to appeal the decision in court is preserved. In addition to determining the existence of liability, arbitration panels also determine the amount of compensation, if any, due the claimant.

Arbitration panel members are often professional arbiters with experience and skill in handling disputes on the subject in question. Through the mutual consent of both parties, panelists are often chosen from lists of qualified arbiters composed by the American Arbitration Association.

There are a number of practical advantages to using screening or arbitration panels for settling private disputes:

- Cases are resolved more quickly than they are in the courtroom, thereby saving litigants time, money, and aggravation.
- The panelists are usually more knowledgeable about technical medical matters than is the typical juror or judge.
- The atmosphere and rules regarding admissibility and relevancy of evidence are more relaxed than those enforced during a trial.
- There seems to be some evidence that arbitration panels are less likely to make excessive, emotionally-induced awards than juries or judges.
- There is less publicity and, therefore, less damage to a physician's reputation.

Since the use of arbitration usually results in less expense to plaintiff and defendant, it offers another advantage to the plaintiff with a legitimate complaint but minimal injuries. Such cases are usually refused by attorneys because the damages recoverable would not even cover the attorney's fees and expenses, given the huge amount of work required to prepare for a medical negligence trial. Therefore, most attorneys will not even consider a case unless the patient was seriously injured, thereby creating the likelihood of a sizable settlement. The availability of arbitration panels enables attorneys to accept as clients those patients with minimal injuries.

There are two types of arbitration agreements—preclaim agreements and postclaim agreements.

1. *Preclaim agreements*: The provider of health care service and the patient agree before service is rendered that if a dispute arises concerning the service, it will be settled through arbitration rather than litigation. Preclaim agreements are offered patients by some hospitals during admission procedures and by a few physicians at the time of the patient's first visit. Preclaim agreements are also a condition for membership in some prepaid medical plans and Health Maintenance Organizations (HMOs).
2. *Postclaim agreements*: These agreements are executed after a dispute arises and both sides agree to resolve it through arbitration rather than litigation.

Some lawyers and constitutional scholars object to preclaim arbitration agreements for one or more of the following reasons:

- No one should be asked to waive his/her right to a jury trial before a dispute arises.
- Most patients who sign preclaim agreements do not understand what they are doing.
- Many patients sign out of fear that not doing so will result in their being refused service at a time when they desperately need it and are in no position to bargain or to go elsewhere for help.

To reduce these objections, efforts recently have been made by health care providers and state legislators to promote a better understanding of the arbitration process.

Many preclaim arbitration agreements now offered patients clearly state that arbitration is an option, not a requirement, and that by selecting that option, the patient waives his/her right to a jury trial.

Most state arbitration laws require that patients be given the right to revoke an arbitration agreement within a reasonable amount of time, usually within 30-60 days of treatment. State laws also stipulate that health care providers may not refuse service because a patient does not agree to arbitrate future disputes.

In the mid- and late-1970s, many states enacted compulsory arbitration laws that mandated arbitration as the means of settling certain types of disputes involving a set amount of money (usually $10,000 or less). Several of these laws have faced and lost constitutional challenges. Some courts have said that the United States Constitution guarantees everyone a right to a trial by jury and that this right cannot be taken away by legislation. Other courts have ruled that certain types of lawsuits cannot be singled out for special or different handling, and that such singling out violates constitutional guarantees of equal protection under the law. A few other statutes requiring compulsory arbitration of malpractice claims have been overturned on technical points, or are currently being challenged.

Holder suggests that the only way to avoid a constitutional challenge to compulsory arbitration laws is to provide the parties with the right to appeal the decision to a trial court for a jury trial. Advocates of compulsory arbitration believe that such a provision would diminish the effectiveness of the arbitration process.

Judicial authorities do not have the same constitutional or legal reservations about postclaim arbitration agreements. As long as both sides knowledgeably and voluntarily agree to arbitrate a dispute after it has arisen, arbitration is considered a fair and just process to settle the matter.

Both arbitration and screening panels are useful supplements and aids to the litigation process. Screening panels have proven effective in discouraging meritless lawsuits and helping plaintiffs with legitimate cases but limited resources. Arbitration is a just, efficient, and relatively inexpensive way of settling some disputes. However, neither arbitration nor screening panels can replace the litigation process that, although sometimes slow and expensive, is the keystone of civil justice in this country.

3. State the two primary goals of joint screening panels.

4. Describe the two types of arbitration agreements.

5. List three advantages of the arbitration process over the litigation process.

PREVENTION OF CONFLICT

The Facility: Quality Assurance/Risk Management

One preventative measure that has been mandated for hospitals for many years for the purpose of providing quality patient care is quality assurance and risk management. The goal of offices, clinics, and other outpatient facilities should be the same—to provide quality patient care.

Quality assurance is the activity of identifying and resolving problems in patient care. It involves ongoing monitoring, evaluation, and improvement of care. Risk management involves efforts to prevent physical and emotional injury to the patients, staff, and visitors, thus protecting the financial assets of the organization by preventing those events that are most likely to lead to liability.

Poor quality creates a risk, which can lead to liability. In order to prevent injury, potential risks must be identified and all incidents monitored. Areas with significant incidents need to be gauged, and corrective measures taken to eliminate these risks. Some common issues for risk management are: appointment delays, lack of sensitivity to patient concerns, unsafe facilities, injection or minor surgery errors, specimen collection and labeling errors, improper procedures for infection control, and lack of documentation of quality control in laboratories (e.g., equipment calibration).

Complete information about quality assurance/risk management can be obtained from the Ambulatory Health Care Standards Manual from the Joint Commission on Accreditation of Health Care Organizations (JCAHO).

Accreditation for outpatient facilities is not mandated, but the standards manual is a superb tool for all facilities.

The Individual: Communication and Care

If one were to analyze the real causes of claims against
health care providers, it would become apparent that the
cause is not necessarily the imperfect or negligent performance of a procedure. Lawsuits are usually triggered by the
absence of a good interpersonal relationship between patient
and health care provider, or the casual, cold, and careless
attitude of support personnel. There is no doubt that each
member of the health care team plays a significant role in
the care given to the patient and in the overall feeling of
confidence and satisfaction that a patient has.

The following general preventative guidelines have
been selected to help associate, assistant, and support personnel in preventing litigation involving themselves and
their employers. There are only six listed; all other ideas
seem to fall into one of the guidelines listed below:

1. Always demonstrate a feeling of genuine concern
   for the welfare of patients. You owe every patient a
   duty of courtesy, consideration, respect, and decent
   treatment. Always use tact and sensitivity when
   dealing with patients and associates.
2. Always respect the confidentiality of the doctor–
   patient relationship. Be careful about when and
   where you discuss patient matters in the office.
   Never discuss patient matters outside the office.
3. Never go beyond the scope and training of your
   field (e.g., do not practice medicine or dentistry).
   Do not perform procedures in which you are not
   adept. Do not hesitate to ask for help or to state that
   you have not been trained in a specific procedure.
4. Always obey federal and state laws as well as local
   ordinances. Do not commit a crime or be an accomplice before or after the fact.
5. Conscientiously follow the procedures designed to
   provide the best of care and to facilitate understanding between health care provider and patient.
   Obtain informed consent, explain procedures, fol-

low up thoroughly, and document carefully. Make sure that the patient understands the diagnosis or condition, the procedure, any instructions, and the reasons for each. Be sure that your patient feels free to ask questions.

6. Keep current on the changes in your particular field, and in the health care field in general. Continuing education is essential.

COMPETENCY CHECK: THREE

6. **Identify the purpose of quality assurance/risk management procedures.**

7. **List some common issues for risk management in an ambulatory care facility.**

8. **True or false: Accreditation of ambulatory care facilities is mandatory.**

9. **Explain the six guidelines listed to help health care practitioners avoid conflict and litigation.**

SUMMARY

Increasingly, health care professionals are being sued by their patients or their patients' families. This chapter, therefore, has presented a review of some of the reasons for this. The litigation process has been described and other ways of resolving disputes have been discussed. Although the alternative methods of resolving conflict between patients and health care providers may be superior to litigation, the best way to prevent conflict is to implement preventative practices.

While there are numerous books and journal articles providing opinions and lists of preventative measures, these concepts and recommendations have been condensed into six preventative guidelines for avoiding litigation and conflict between health care professionals and patients. Basically, a genuine concern for the welfare of every patient and the conscientious and careful performance of all procedures is probably the best defense and the best method of providing quality health care.

When you have finished reading this chapter, complete the corresponding chapter in your workbook and then proceed to Chapter 14.

14

Medical Ethics and Bioethical Issues

Although this book is concerned primarily with medical law, medical ethics—itself the subject for a book—must concurrently be viewed in the light of its relationship to the law.

By common definition, law is a rule of conduct enforced by a controlling authority; a code of ethics is an established set of moral principles and values. Together they provide legal and moral guidelines for the care and treatment of patients, for relationships between health and allied health professionals, and for the relationships of all health care providers with the public.

The American Medical Association and many other professional organizations have developed, and their members adhere to, specific codes of ethics. These are the focus of this chapter.

The Principles of Medical Ethics established by the American Medical Association state the primary goals of the medical profession. These principles are interpreted by AMA's Judicial Council through its periodic publication of *Current Opinions of the Judicial Council,* which provides guidelines for applying the principles in everyday medical practice.

Many other health care practitioners are duty-bound to uphold the principles established by the American Medical Association, just as they are duty-bound to uphold the code of ethics developed by their own organizations.

Both the AMA's Principles of Medical Ethics and the Oath of Hippocrates are presented, interpreted, and discussed in this chapter. They have been included to provide the groundwork for a discussion of the relationship between law and ethics and also to provide a springboard for an in-depth study of the subject of ethics in the health care professions.

BACKGROUND

While each of us is subject to law, each of us also has an unwritten code that guides our personal behavior. In addition, most of us also belong to groups of people that set standards of behavior for members of the group. This is especially common in the health professions.

The purpose of law is to help regulate the conduct of individuals. The purpose of codes of professional ethics is to provide a guide to responsible professional behavior. Both are ways of integrating the needs, goals, and behaviors of individuals with the needs, goals, and behaviors of the larger group. There are, however, some important differences between law and ethics.

One difference is in degree. It is often said that laws state the lowest standards of conduct that society will permit, while ethics state the highest standards and ideals to which all should aspire. Ethical standards, especially professional standards, are usually greater, but are never less than or contrary to legal standards.

Another difference is in scope. From the discussion of law earlier in this book, you know that legal standards apply equally to all citizens and are established and enforced through government. Ethical standards, however, are established by individuals or by organized groups of people who share a common interest in a subject—be it based on religion, business, or profession. These individuals or groups establish a code of behavior applicable only to themselves or to members of the group. Being censured, suspended, or expelled from membership is the usual punishment for not adhering to a code of ethics, with expulsion being the most severe.

HISTORY OF MEDICAL ETHICS

Throughout its history, the medical profession has subscribed to ethical principles based on certain fundamentals:

- The individual patient's welfare is of prime concern.

- Information acquired by doctors during the course of treatment must be kept confidential.
- Medical privileges must not be abused.
- The doctor has a duty to instruct.

Figure 14-A. The Oath of Hippocrates

I swear by Apollo, the physician, and Aesculapius and health and all-heal and all the Gods and Goddesses that, according to my ability and judgment, I will keep this oath and stipulation:

To reckon him who taught me this art equally dear to me as my parents, to share my substance with him and relieve his necessities if required, to regard his offspring as on the same footing with my own brothers, and to teach them this art if they should wish to learn it, without fee or stipulation, and that by precept, lecture and every mode of instruction, I will impart a knowledge of the art to my own sons and to those of my teachers, and to disciples bound by a stipulation and oath, according to the law of medicine, but to none others.

I will follow that method of treatment which, according to my ability and judgment, I consider for the benefit of my patients, and abstain from whatever is deleterious and mischievous. I will give no deadly medicine to anyone if asked, nor suggest any such counsel; furthermore, I will not give to a woman an instrument to produce abortion.

With purity and with holiness I will pass my life and practice my art. I will not cut a person who is suffering from a stone, but will leave this to be done by practitioners of this work. Into whatever houses I enter I will go into them for the benefit of the sick and will abstain from every voluntary act of mischief and corruption; and further from the seduction of females or males, bond or free.

Whatever, in connection with my professional practice, or not in connection with it, I may see or hear in the lives of men which ought not to be spoken abroad I will not divulge, as reckoning that all such should be kept secret.

While I continue to keep this oath unviolated may it be granted to me to enjoy life and the practice of the art, respected by all men at all times but should I trespass and violate this oath, may the reverse be my lot.

Although expressed differently through the ages, these fundamentals have guided doctors from the time of the Babylonians to modern time. The Oath of Hippocrates, written probably in the 5th Century B.C. (the exact time has never been determined), expresses these sentiments and remains the bedrock of medical ethics today. Upon graduation from medical school, many medical students swear to abide by this oath, a modern version of which appears as Figure 14-A. An English doctor, Thomas Percival, made another significant contribution to the history of medical ethics in 1803 when he published a *Code of Medical Ethics*, which was widely circulated and accepted.

The American Medical Association, established in 1847, had two subjects on the agenda of its first substantive meeting: (1) standards of medical education; and (2) the adoption of a code of medical ethics. The Code of Ethics, adopted in 1847, was based primarily on Percival's code. It remained essentially the same until 1957 when it was shortened and rearranged into a preamble and ten short sections.

In 1980, the Code was revised to clarify and update the language, to eliminate reference to gender, and to seek a proper balance between professional standards and contemporary legal standards in our changing society. The latest version of the Principles of Medical Ethics is reprinted in Figure 14-B. It consists of a preamble and seven sections.You should read them carefully before proceeding.

Some of the basic points underlying the Principles of Medical Ethics are subsequently restated and emphasized.

- Providing competent medical service is the paramount objective of the medical profession; all other objectives, including financial return and scientific advancement, are subordinate concerns.
- The right of free choice is basic to the practice of medicine in this country. Patients are free to choose a doctor or a preferred system of medical care, and doctors are free, except in emergencies, to choose patients and the circumstances under which they wish to practice.

- The Principles of Medical Ethics apply to all physicians, regardless of the nature and structure of their practice. It makes no difference whether the doctor is in a solo, partnership, group, or clinic practice, or whether the doctor is employed by another doctor or organization.

Figure 14-B. Principles of Medical Ethics

Preamble: *The medical profession has long subscribed to a body of ethical statements developed primarily for the benefit of the patient. As a member of this profession, a physician must recognize responsibility not only to patients, but also to society, to other health professionals, and to self. The following Principles adopted by the American Medical Association are not laws, but standards of conduct which define the essentials of honorable behavior for the physician.*

I. A physician shall be dedicated to providing competent medical service with compassion and respect for human dignity.

II. A physician shall deal honestly with patients and colleagues, and strive to expose those physicians deficient in character or competence, or who engage in fraud or deception.

III. A physician shall respect the law and also recognize a responsibility to seek changes in those requirements which are contrary to the best interests of the patient.

IV. A physician shall respect the rights of patients, of colleagues, and of other health professionals, and shall safeguard patient confidences within the constraints of the law.

V. A physician shall continue to study, apply, and advance scientific knowledge, make relevant information available to patients, colleagues, and the public, obtain consultation, and use the talents of other health professionals when indicated.

VI. A physician shall, in the provision of appropriate patient care, except in emergencies, be free to choose whom to serve, with whom to associate, and the environment in which to provide medical services.

VII. A physician shall recognize a responsibility to participate in activities contributing to an improved community.

- A chief purpose of the Principles is to discourage practices that could exploit patients or that could interfere with the patient's right to choose a doctor or a preferred system of medical care.
- Local and state medical societies are autonomous organizations that may impose restrictions differing from those established by the national association.

MEDICAL ETHICS FOR DOCTORS

As noted earlier, the American Medical Association's Judicial Council is charged with interpreting the Principles of Medical Ethics and with guiding their application in the general practice of medicine. It is also charged with expressing opinions related to ethics in specific clinical situations.

Ethics in General Practice

A number of topics addressed by the Council have interest for, and relevance to, allied health professionals. Some of the most pertinent are discussed in the following pages.

Fees. The AMA Judicial Council has remarked on several matters related to doctors' fees. Many of the remarks reiterate and reinforce the Council's opinion that a doctor's medical practice is not a commercial enterprise where the primary objective is profit, but a professional practice where the primary consideration is patient welfare.

Doctors' fees for medical services should be reasonable, and never excessive. Factors considered in whether a fee is reasonable include:

- Difficulty and uniqueness of the service provided, plus the time, skill, and experience required.
- Fees charged by other doctors in the same locale for the same service.
- Results.
- Relationship between doctor and patient.
- Doctor's reputation and ability.
- Total amount of charges.

At patients' requests, doctors should complete simple health insurance claim forms without charge. Whether to charge for completing complex forms should be determined by local custom and individual circumstances.

Charging patients for missed appointments or appointments not cancelled within twenty-four hours is not encouraged as a routine practice, but it is not unethical if the patient is notified of the policy in advance. Before a charge is levied, individual consideration must be given each patient and the circumstances surrounding the late cancellation or no-show.

Charging a distinct fee for the procedure of admitting a patient to the hospital is unethical.

Charging or accepting a fee for referring a patient to another individual or agency is unethical.

Doctors' fees should be fixed, although they may be reduced for patients with financial difficulties. Fees contingent upon the outcome of a patient's claim against a third party are improper. A doctor's fee should reflect the value of the service provided, not the outcome of a settlement.

Doctors may make use of doctors' lien laws, provided the fee is fixed and not contingent on settlement.

If a doctor refers a patient to a laboratory or uses the services of one, the laboratory should bill the patient directly. If this is not possible and the laboratory bills the doctor, the doctor may in turn bill the patient provided the laboratory services and fees are itemized.

When a doctor observes, directs, supervises and assumes responsibility for services provided a patient by a resident, the doctor may bill the patient for those services. Who actually performs the surgery or procedure must never be misrepresented.

Advertising. Doctors may advertise as they wish, provided they do not use practices that may tend to mislead or deceive the public. A doctor may advertise in any communications medium provided the message or communication does not omit significant information; contain inaccurate, untrue, or misleading information; or otherwise deceive or mislead.

The message may include the educational background of the doctor, how fees are determined, payment plans or options, and any other information a reasonable person would consider relevant in selecting a doctor's services. Statements implying that the doctor's skills or remedies are unique, exclusive, or superior should be avoided, because they may create unjustified expectations.

In accordance with federal regulations, the doctor whose services are being advertised will be held responsible for the accuracy and truthfulness of content in the communication. The same rules apply to commercial communications concerning doctors' groups, partnerships, etc.

Medical Records. With regard to medical records:

- Doctors have an ethical obligation to protect the confidentiality of patients' medical records. This obligation extends to medical information stored on computers. The AMA Judicial Council has developed some guidelines to help doctors and computer service organizations protect the confidentiality of the information stored in computer databases. Highlights of these guidelines include:

  1. Both doctor and patient should know if and where confidential medical information about the patient is stored on computers.
  2. Persons and organizations with access to the database should be identified.
  3. Information that identifies a patient should never be released by the service bureau without the doctor's and patient's express approval. Information should be released only to individuals and organizations with a legitimate need and use for the information and only for the specific purpose for which the information is requested. Such release of confidential medical information should be limited to the specific time frame requested and should not be released to other individuals or organizations.

4. Procedures for erasing old or inaccurate data from the data base should be set, and both patient and doctor should be notified before and after information has been destroyed.
5. A doctor's computerized patient records should never be mixed with those of other clients of the computer service bureau.
6. Access to the data base must be limited to authorized individuals.
7. The computer service bureau must closely monitor employees to ensure only authorized personnel have access to the facility and records.

- Doctors have an ethical duty to release information from a patient's medical records when required by law or by the request or consent of the patient.
- When a doctor decides to retire or move, he/she should notify patients in the active file, suggest they select another doctor, and offer to make available a copy of their records to the succeeding doctor. To transfer a patient's records without proper consent is a violation of the doctor-patient confidence. (For their own legal protection, retiring doctors should keep original patient records indefinitely, or at least until the statutory period for filing professional liability suits has expired.)
- When a partnership is dissolved or a doctor-employee terminates his/her relationship with a group or clinic practice, patients' interests in their records should be served. A doctor who needs to review a prior patient's records should have the privilege of doing so, with the patient's consent.

COMPETENCY CHECK: ONE

1. True or false: The primary objective of the medical profession is the advancement of scientific knowledge.

2. True or false: Ethical standards of professional conduct and responsibility may exceed, but are never less than or contrary to those required by law.

3. **True or False: Protecting the confidentiality of patient records stored in computer bases is the responsibility of the computer service agency, not the doctor.**

Relationships with Others

Most doctors refer patients to other health care professionals and related organizations on a daily basis. A doctor should make a referral whenever it would benefit the patient. Further, the doctor should refer patients only to those persons or organizations by whom he/she can confidently expect the required services to be performed competently, scientifically, and legally. With these overall considerations in mind, let's consider a variety of relationships that the typical doctor has with other health care personnel.

Doctors. A doctor may, and indeed should, refer a patient to another doctor whenever it would be in the patient's best interests. As a courtesy, the doctor to whom the patient is referred should periodically inform the referring doctor of the patient's progress.

A doctor may, and indeed should, request a consultation whenever it would be in the patient's best interest. A consultation is a request for another doctor's opinion. The doctor making the request remains in charge of treating the patient. When a patient is sent to a consultant, the doctor-in-charge should inform the consultant of the patient's relevant history, the current treatment plan, and the medical opinion of the doctor-in-charge. The consultant should send the doctor-in-charge a summary of his/her findings and opinions soon after the patient has been seen.

The AMA Judicial Council states that for one surgeon to permit another to operate on the first surgeon's patient without the patient's consent is a serious violation of ethical principles and also is a violation of the legal requirement to have the patient's informed consent. This practice, sometimes referred to as "ghost surgery," violates the patient's rights to choose a doctor, as well as the contractual agreement between doctor and patient.

It is a common and ethical practice for a patient's surgeon to hire an assistant or to ask a resident to assist with an operation. As long as the patient's surgeon is the operating surgeon and any financial arrangement between surgeon and assistant is disclosed to the patient, the practice is in accord with ethical principles and sound medical practice.

However, if the patient's surgeon plans to guide a resident or assistant surgeon during the operation, the resident or assistant must be considered the "operating surgeon." Thus, the patient must agree to the substitution, in advance and in writing, for the practice to be considered ethical.

Nondoctor health care providers. A doctor may refer a patient to nondoctor providers of health care services whenever it would be in the patient's best interests. In all referrals, the doctor must be confident of the competence of the person or organization to whom he/she is referring.

Nonmedical personnel. *Patient representatives.* A doctor's duty to his/her patient often exceeds providing medical services.

> In many instances, the peculiar knowledge and attainments of the doctor are indispensable to patients or others in the administration of business and government and in the usual conduct of certain daily affairs. When this knowledge, acquired through the course of the doctor-patient relationship, is necessary to enable the patient to obtain his just due, the doctor should make it available for the patient's benefit under proper conditions.[1]

A doctor has an ethical obligation to cooperate with the patient's attorney and insurance company, to cite just two examples. As a general rule, doctors should comply with all patient-authorized requests for information concerning the patient's health status.

Media representatives. Representatives of the communications media often ask doctors for information on specific patients, as well as for information on subjects of general medical and public health interest. The Principles of Medical Ethics encourage doctors to cooperate with media representatives in accordance with ethical and legal considerations.

Clearly, a doctor may not directly or indirectly reveal a patient's condition to the media without the consent of the patient or the patient's authorized representative.

4. Give two examples of representatives to whom patients
    commonly authorize release of medical information.

BIOETHICAL ISSUES: ETHICS IN CLINICAL SITUATIONS

As stated, the Judicial Council expresses its opinion on current medical procedures and social issues. As you will see,
these opinions are based on certain fundamental ethical
standards that have remained constant through time:

1. the paramount importance of the individual
    patient's welfare;
2. the right of patients to choose their physician; and
3. the right of physicians to choose their patients.

Scarce Resources

The questions surrounding the issue of scarce resources are
complex and formidable: Who will get the next available
kidney? Which patient should get the last bed in the inten-
sive care unit? If there is one cardiac arrest team and two
patients in cardiac arrest, which one should the team attend?
Who will decide who receives scarce resources? How will
these decisions be made? What will the criteria be for these
decisions?

Allocation of Health Resources

In addition to inherently scarce resources such as organs
and ICU beds, a broader spectrum of health care resources
may become scarce, then rationed, and finally allocated.

    Adequate health care for all has been a concern for
many years. The federal government attempted to address
the problem of greater access to quality care with Medicare
and Medicaid legislation.

    Oregon was the first state to face the fact that the state
could not afford unlimited health care for all citizens. How

should the state resources be used? Should $40,000 of public funds be used for a transplant for one child, or should that money be used to provided prenatal and well-baby care for two-hundred women and their children?

The Health Services Commission was created by the Oregon legislature. Discussions were conducted throughout the state with medical, social, and legal professionals, with legislators and local government officials, and with the public. A system of rationing was devised for funding a prioritized list of conditions and health care. Other states are studying the Oregon Plan and considering what they are going to do to stretch resources and provide care for as many people as possible.

Berlex Laboratories of Wayne, New Jersey, has received FDA approval for a drug to treat multiple sclerosis, but Berlex only has enough of the drug to treat 20,000 patients, which is approximately a fifth of those who could potentially benefit. In an effort to distribute the drug fairly, Berlex has organized a computerized lottery to dispense the drug. Patients will be chosen randomly and payment will be on a sliding scale for those who can pay and free to the rest.

While some medical ethicists think that this approach is reasonable, some difficult questions have been raised. Is this really the best and the most equitable way to allocate a very scarce resource?

Judicial Council Opinion

The AMA strongly opposes rationing plans that would limit beneficial care to patients on the basis of cost. If health care were to be limited or denied on the basis of cost, the care being denied would, therefore, become a limited resource and allocation criteria applied.

Five factors relating to health care need should be taken into account when allocating organs or other scarce resources—ICU beds or bypass surgery. The factors are: (1) the likelihood of benefit to the patient, (2) the impact of treatment in improving the quality of the patient's life, (3) the duration of benefit, (4) the urgency of the patient's con-

dition (i.e. how close is the patient to death), and in some cases, (5) the amount of resources required for successful treatment. The criteria are not to be applied in an arbitrary manner nor one criterion given precedence over the others and allowed to serve as a priority principle.

Factors that are considered ethically unacceptable in allocating scarce resources are (1) ability to pay, (2) past use of resources, (3) contribution of the patient to society (social worth), (4) perceived obstacles to treatment (patients with multiple diseases or language barriers, alcohol and drug abusers, the indigent, the uneducated), and (5) contribution of the patient to his or her own medical condition.

Organ Donation

Judicial Council Opinion

Voluntary donation of organs in appropriate circumstances is to be encouraged. It is not ethical to participate in a procedure to enable a donor to receive payment, other than for the reimbursement of expenses necessarily incurred in connection with removal.

ORGAN TRANSPLANTATION

Issues and Potential Issues

Many doubts and questions surround the issue of organ transplants. Who should receive the next available organ? Should candidates be ranked on a national or local level? Should candidates be allowed to seek media coverage and possibly receive an organ before candidates with more critical need? When should a patient be restricted from receiving multiple transplants?

Should couples conceive in order to provide organs or tissue for a sibling or parent and, if so, will a fetus that is considered incompatible be aborted? Should fetal tissue be used for transplants?

Should brain-dead accident victims be kept alive until relatives are located and permission obtained for organ donation. Should the family then be billed for the life-maintenance costs?

Should it be legal to buy organs? The transplant of kidneys from live donors is so commonplace among the poor in Egypt and India that officials are alarmed. Although the practice is considered immoral and sales of kidneys are condemned, the transactions are not illegal. Furthermore, it is feared that any ban on sales would only send the practice underground and place both donor and recipient in an increasingly dangerous situation.

Judicial Council Opinion

The same concern for their patients' welfare that guides physicians in all patient relationships should guide them in transplant procedures. The Judicial Council has developed special guidelines for physicians in this area:

- *The rights of both the donor and the recipient must be protected equally, and scientific advancement must be of secondary importance to the welfare of the patient.*
- *Prospective organ donors must be offered the same quality of care and the same treatment alternatives offered patients with similar injuries and diseases.*
- *When a vital organ is to be transplanted, the death of the donor must not be determined by the recipient's physician. At least one other physician must determine it, using currently-accepted scientific procedures.*
- *The informed consents of both donor and recipient or their legal representatives are mandatory.*
- *Transplant procedures should be undertaken only: (1) by qualified physicians, (2) in adequate facilities, and (3) after alternative procedures are carefully evaluated.*

Distribution of organs should be allocated following the United Network of Organ Sharing (UNOS) guidelines.

Geographical priorities in the allocation of organs should be prohibited except when transportation of organs would threaten their suitability for transplantation.

Anencephalic Infants as Organ Donors

Judicial Council Opinion

Retrieval and transplantation of the organs of an anencephalic infant is ethically permissible in accordance with determination of death guidelines. Physician may provide ventilator assistance and other medical therapies necessary to sustain organ perfusion and viability until such time that the determination of death can be made.

Medical Applications of Fetal Tissue Transplantation

Judicial Council Opinion

The degree to which the decision to have an abortion might be influenced by the decision to donate the postmortem tissue of the fetus is the primary ethical concern. There are several guidelines to be followed in this instance. The decision to have an abortion must be made before any discussion of the use of fetal tissue is discussed. There is to be no payment for the tissue, and the donor may not choose the recipient. The health care personnel involved in the abortion may not benefit from the tissue transplantation. There must be informed consent of both donor and recipient. Guidelines for clinical investigation and organ transplants should be followed.

COMPETENCY CHECK: THREE

5. True or false. An AMA Judicial Council Opinion states that the AMA strongly opposes rationing plans that would limit beneficial care to patients on the basis of cost.

244 Health Care Law and Ethics

6. True or false. According to a Judicial Council Opinion, it is ethical to make decisions about allocating scarce resources on the basis of the patient's contribution to society.

HUMAN REPRODUCTION AND THE FAMILY

"The family" has undergone a radical change in the past decade. Besides stepparents, foster parents, adoptive parents, and custodial grandparents, there are many nontraditional families. Thanks to surrogate mothers, sperm and ova donors, and new technologies, infertile couples, postmenopausal women, single people, and homosexual couples can bear children.

If there is a high risk of having a child with a genetic disease, it is now possible to choose not to reproduce, to accept the risk of having a child with a genetic anomaly, to undergo prenatal diagnosis and abort a fetus, to use one of the artificial reproductive technologies, or to adopt a child.

Conception

Recent technological advances have made it possible to achieve parenthood through in vitro fertilization, GIFT (gamete intrafallopian transfer), artificial insemination, use of a surrogate womb, and donor eggs or sperm.

Artificial Insemination. The procedure of artificial insemination may be done with sperm provided by the woman's husband or with sperm provided by a donor. When the husband provides the sperm, the procedure is known as AIH (Artificial Insemination Homologous), and there is no legal question about the legitimacy of the biological offspring.

When a donor provides the sperm, the procedure is known as AID (Artificial Insemination Donor). This procedure has raised some legal questions about the legitimacy and rights of the offspring.

In states that have addressed the issue statutorily, a child born to a married woman and conceived through AID is considered legitimate, provided the woman's husband consented to the procedure. A few states require that the husband's consent to the AID procedure be in writing. Even in the absence of such a state law, a doctor would want to discuss the procedure with a patient's husband and obtain his written consent. The wife's written consent should also be obtained. In addition, many authorities recommend obtaining the written consent of the donor and his wife (if any).

Doctors must use care in screening prospective donors to ensure genetic compatibility with the recipient, as well as to eliminate donors with medical or genetic problems. Further, the donor should not be known by the prospective parent(s), nor should his identity ever be revealed.

Likewise, the identity of the recipient and her husband should never be revealed to the donor. Records documenting the procedure must be kept, but extra precautions should be taken to protect the confidentiality of the records.

In vitro fertilization and GIFT. In vitro fertilization is the process in which the ovum of the woman is fertilized by the sperm of the man "in glass"—in a test tube or culture dish. After the ovum is fertilized, it is transferred to a container for three to six days to mature. It is then transplanted to the uterus of the woman (mother), and the pregnancy continues as usual.

The procedure has offered couples who have been infertile due to damage or obstruction of the fallopian tubes or oviducts the opportunity to produce children. There have not been many ethical questions regarding in vitro fertilization involving a couple. The ethical and legal concerns arise from the use of donor sperm or donor ova, or when unused zygotes (fertilized ova) are used for research.

Gamete intrafallopian transfer (GIFT) is accomplished by administering hormones to increase production of eggs. Then, during ovulation, the doctor removes eggs with a laparoscope. The eggs mature in the laboratory. The eggs and the partner's concentrated sperm are then placed in a catheter with air and inserted through a laparoscope into the woman's fallopian tube. A woman must have one open fallopian tube in order to benefit from GIFT.

Judicial Council Opinion

Professional ethics do not prohibit artificial human insemination. The informed consent of the woman seeking artificial insemination and her husband is necessary. A child conceived and born through artificial insemination (AIH) has the same legal rights as a child conceived and born naturally. Extra precautions should be taken to ensure the confidentiality of the procedure and of related records. Health care providers who are personally opposed to conception by artificial means are not obligated to participate in procedures.

Any fertilized egg that has the potential for human life and that will be implanted in the uterus of a woman should not be subjected to laboratory research.

Pre-embryos obtained through in vitro fertilization that are not used at the time may be frozen in case future implantations are necessary or desired. Agreements deciding the disposition of frozen pre-embryos in the event of divorce or other changes in circumstances are subject to legal and ethical challenge. The following guidelines should be observed:

1. The man and woman who provided the gametes (eggs and sperm) should have control over the frozen embryos—whether they should be used by them, donated to others, or destroyed (but not sold).
2. Research should be permitted in accordance with the guidelines on fetal research.
3. The providers of the eggs and the sperm should have equal say in the use of the pre-embryos.

Surrogacy. A surrogate is a woman who agrees to carry a fetus until term for a couple. The surrogate may be artificially inseminated with the sperm of the father or with the fertilized ovum of the couple. There is a contractual agreement in which the surrogate mother agrees to relinquish all rights to the infant at birth, and the couple pays the woman's expenses and a fee.

Issues and Potential Issues

Court cases have made apparent some of the issues concerning surrogacy. Surrogate mothers in some cases have refused to give the infant to the contracted couple. Questions become complicated when there is a surrogate mother who carried the fetus that was the result of an ovum taken from the woman (wife) and fertilized by the sperm of the man (husband). The questions become even more involved when the sperm of the man (husband) fertilizes the ovum of the surrogate. How many "parents" does that child have? What happens if the ovum was from a donor (maybe a relative of the wife), the sperm was from the husband, and the surrogate carried the fetus? How many "parents" are there, and who are the custodial "parents"?

Judicial Council Opinion

Surrogacy does not, for various ethical, social and legal reasons, represent a satisfactory reproductive alternative for people who wish to become parents.

Prenatal Screening—Genetic Counseling

The Human Genome Project is expected to help identify and cure disease at the genetic level and to broaden the understanding of genetic influences on human behavior.

Prenatal genetic screening is an emerging technique. Currently, prenatal screening is performed through blood testing, amniocentesis or chorionic villi sampling during gestation, or—in artificial reproductive techniques— through examination of a pre-embryo. Down's syndrome, hemophilia, phenylketonuria, sickle cell anemia, and Tay-Sachs disease can be predicted with some certainty.

Genetic manipulation is the alteration, replacement, or repair of an undesired gene. It may become possible to correct single gene defects. Promising results have been achieved with adenosine deaminase deficiency, cystic fibrosis, and melanoma.

Issues and Potential Issues

Genetic screening and gene therapy represent a significant step forward in the ability to diagnose, treat, and eliminate genetically caused disorders, but they are costly and the benefits may be available only to a small portion of the population. While gene manipulation can be used to avoid mental retardation, should it be used to control intelligence? Discriminatory practices can be foreseen as a result of genetic screening and manipulation. (Sex selection is an obvious potential concern.) Will only the more affluent be able to afford this technology, and therefore be healthier? Will specific behavior patterns be eliminated? Who decides? People from different cultural backgrounds view and define health, sickness, and treatment differently. Will they be excluded from the benefits, and therefore more vulnerable to elimination?

Judicial Council Opinion

Physicians should promote informed reproductive choices by counseling prospective parents on the availability and role of prenatal genetic screening, including reasons for and against screening and the appropriate uses of genetic testing. Physicians could participate in genetic selection to prevent, cure, or treat genetic disease. A number of factors need to be considered: (1) the severity of the disease, (2) the probability of its occurrence, (3) the age of onset, and (4) the time of gestation at which selection would occur. It would not be ethical to engage in genetic selection on the basis of non-disease-causing characteristics or traits.

COMPETENCY CHECK: FOUR

7. **True or false. There are no legal questions about the legitimacy and rights of the offspring produced by Artificial Insemination Donor (AID).**

8. **True or false. In vitro fertilization is a process in which the ovum of a woman is fertilized by the sperm of the man "in glass."**

Abortion

On January 22, 1973, the United States Supreme Court made two decisions that are as controversial today as they were then.

In the case of *Roe v Wade*, the court stipulated the conditions under which a state had the authority to regulate nontherapeutic abortions. In that decision, which liberalized abortion law throughout the country, the court said:

1. During the first thirteen weeks of fetal gestation, a state has no authority whatsoever to regulate abortions, except to require that the procedure be performed by a licensed doctor. During a woman's first trimester of pregnancy, the decision to abort belongs to her and to her doctor.
2. During the second trimester of pregnancy (defined as beginning after the first thirteen weeks and ending just before the fetus becomes viable), a state may establish reasonable regulations designed to enhance maternal health, such as stipulating that a second trimester abortion be performed only under certain medical conditions. The state has no right to prohibit abortions during this period.
3. During the third trimester of pregnancy, which begins when the fetus becomes viable (usually between the twenty-fourth and twenty-eighth week of pregnancy), a state may regulate and even prohibit nontherapeutic abortions. This part of the decision is based on the Supreme Court's belief that only after a fetus becomes viable does the state have the right to take steps to protect its life.

On that same date—January 22, 1973—the Supreme Court decided the case of *Doe v Bolton*. In that decision, the court said that a state could not impose procedural conditions that unfairly restricted a woman's right to choose an abortion or a doctor's right to exercise good medical judgment.

Specifically, the court said that a state could not: (1) establish residency requirements; (2) require the written concurrence of doctors in addition to the patient's doctor; or (3) require hospital approval or the approval of a court or of a law enforcement officer.

In the *Doe v Bolton* case, the court ruled that states can grant medical personnel the right to refuse to participate in abortion procedures on moral or religious grounds, and that states can require the keeping of certain abortion records which must be provided or made available to the state.

Since the *Roe* and *Doe* decisions in 1973, the United States Supreme Court and some of the federal appellate courts have clarified and limited these two landmark decisions. A thorough treatment of all the abortion decisions since 1973 is beyond the scope of this text. Regardless of what the courts decide, the underlying ethical issues remain.

Technological advancements providing artificial life-support systems at earlier stages of fetal development are straining previously held concepts of fetal viability. Since a state may prohibit abortion after a fetus becomes viable, the question arises: What will happen when a woman's right to an abortion collides with the state's claim that a fetus is viable, given the assistance of artificial extrauterine life-support systems?

This area of health law and ethics remains difficult for health care professionals because the law is often ambiguous and has been changing rapidly. The only safe course for medical personnel involved in this area of health care is to monitor closely the latest laws within their state, to adhere to them strictly, to make sure informed consents are obtained from all patients, and to keep good medical records of all procedures.

Judicial Council Opinion

Physicians may ethically perform abortions in accordance with applicable laws and sound medical practice. A physician personally opposed to abortion is not obligated to accept a patient requesting one.

Fetal Tissue Research

Judicial Council Opinion

Ethically, health care providers may participate in fetal research if the activities are part of an acceptably designed program to produce data which are scientifically valid and significant. The research must conform with the accepted standards of scientific research. Clinical studies with animals and nongravid humans must precede the fetal research. The fetus should never receive physical abuse; the fetus should receive the same care and concern as one in a nonresearch setting. No fees are collected. The project is reviewed by a committee or advisory board. All federal and state laws must be observed. A written, fully-informed consent must be received from the gravid woman or her legal representative.

Sterilization

Sexual sterilization is the procedure of rendering a person incapable of reproducing children. The customary procedure for sterilizing men is by vasectomy—closing the *vas deferens* by either tying off or excising a portion of it. It is a relatively simple procedure, and may be performed in a doctor's office under local anesthesia. It is sometimes reversible.

The procedure most frequently used to sterilize women is tubal ligation. The medical term "salpingectomy" is sometimes used to denote the procedure; it means the partial or total excision of the fallopian tubes. This procedure is more complicated than a vasectomy and is generally performed in a hospital, sometimes in the outpatient department.

There are other medical procedures that result in sexual sterilization—removal of the uterus and/or ovaries and removal of the testes—but these procedures are performed to treat disease, with sterilization a side effect rather than the goal.

Therapeutic Sterilization

The term therapeutic sterilization is used to denote the sterilization procedure when it is performed to preserve the life or health of a patient. It is occasionally done to prevent a woman from becoming pregnant or when a pregnancy would endanger her life or health (mental and emotional as well as physical). At other times, the loss of reproductive power is incidental to the primary purpose of the procedure, such as removing a diseased uterus or removing a prostate gland to prevent the spread of cancer.

There are no special laws governing the performance of therapeutic sterilization, other than a few statutes authorizing it or stipulating that it is not contrary to public policy. However, because the ability to reproduce is so important to many people, the doctor must make sure that eliminating this ability is absolutely necessary and that the patient fully understands and consents to what is to be done. Obtaining another medical opinion or a consultation is the recommended course of action in many circumstances.

Voluntary, Elective, or Contraceptive Sterilization

The terms voluntary, elective, and contraceptive (often used interchangeably) denote the type of sterilization the goal of which is permanent prevention of conception. While some people object to sterilization for purposes of convenience, it is now lawful in every state.

All states have laws stipulating that the procedures be performed by licensed doctors and in licensed facilities. A minimum age—18 or 21 (or the age required for marriage)—has been set in every state. Some states require that the patient be given a detailed written explanation of the procedure and that there be a waiting period of approximately thirty days between that explanation and the performance of the procedure.

Since the vasectomy procedure has a failure rate of approximately 4% and the tubal ligation procedure a failure rate of about 1.7%, doctors should not guarantee patients that they will be sterile after either procedure. In fact, the consent form authorizing the procedure should include the statement that the doctor does not guarantee sterility. The importance of postvasectomy sperm counts should be explained to male patients.

Physicians may refuse to perform contraceptive sterilization procedures on religious or moral grounds. Most states have enacted conscience laws permitting health care professionals and private hospitals receiving no public funds to refuse to perform sterilization procedures for religious or moral objections without fear of legal recriminations.

Adoption

The role of most doctors in adoption procedures is related to the medical evaluation and/or care of the prospective adoptee and, in some cases, to the medical evaluation and/or care of the natural mother or adoptive parents as well. Most legal authorities strongly recommend that physicians restrict their participation in adoption procedures to subjects requiring their medical expertise. Still, some physicians and other health care professionals agree to serve as intermediaries in adoption procedures.

Many states only authorize placement of children for adoption by an approved or licensed agency. These states believe that reputable adoption agencies are the best way to place a child—best for the child, best for the child's natural parents (particularly the mother), and best for the adopting parents.

Agency adoption is considered best for the child because it is more likely to ensure a suitable, secure home. Agency adoption is best for the natural parents because it provides legal safeguards, personal and medical counseling, and assurance that the child will be with loving parents. And finally, agency adoption is best for the adopting parents who can be confident that they will receive a healthy child and that their legal interests will be protected once the placement is made. For all these reasons and more, doctors usually refer patients interested in some phase of adoption to a reputable adoption agency.

If a doctor agrees to act as an intermediary in an adoption situation, the doctor should consult an attorney for legal advice and assistance.

COMPETENCY CHECK: FIVE

9. True or false. According to *Roe v. Wade* and subsequent court cases, a state may not prohibit nontherapeutic abortions during the third trimester.

10. True or false. A vasectomy is always reversible.

11. True or false. Most states permit health care professionals to refuse to perform contraceptive sterilization on religious or moral grounds.

RELATIONSHIP WITH PATIENT

Patient Information

Judicial Council Opinion

Physicians are required to make relevant information available to patients, colleagues, and the public. Physicians must appropriately and adequately explain to their patients the nature and purpose of recommended or prescribed treatment.

Neglect of Patient

Judicial Council Opinion

Physicians are free to choose whom they will serve. However, physicians should respond to any request for assistance in an emergency. Once having undertaken a case, a physician should not neglect the patient, nor withdraw from the case without giving notice to the patient or to the patient's representative sufficiently in advance to permit the patient to secure another attendant.

Unnecessary Services

Judicial Council Opinion

A physician should never prescribe or provide unnecessary services or refer a patient for unnecessary services.

Costs of Health Care

Judicial Council Opinion

Physicians should always be conscious of costs, and not prescribe unnecessary services or medications. The doctor's first concern must always be the welfare of the patient. A physician may participate, individually or through a medical organization, in policy making with respect to social issues affecting health care.

HIV, ARC, and AIDS

Issues and Potential Issues

There are innumerable issues and potential issues involving AIDS: Do victims of sexual battery have the right to require HIV testing? Do they have the right to know the results of prior or current tests? Should all individuals treated for sexually transmitted disease be tested for HIV? Is confidentiality absolute?

Who should treat AIDS patients? Should health care providers be allowed to refuse to care for AIDS patients? Who decides?

A physician may disclose certain confidential AIDS information to the public health department. Statutes allow public health officials to notify and warn partners of possible exposure to AIDS. One of the most difficult issues for health care providers is the disclosure of HIV-positive information to a known partner of the patient. In many states, a physician may inform and warn partners of HIV-related information, but ethical and legal problems occur when the known partner is not a patient of the physician who is caring for the HIV-positive patient.

There are many concerns revolving around the disclosure of HIV, ARC, and AIDS information. The fear of discrimination has created a strong sentiment for nondisclosure of results. Another great concern involves the undermining of the patient-physician confidential relationship. If patients cannot trust the confidentiality of their disclosures, what effect will this have on the patient-physician relationship? What effect will it have on the spread of the HIV virus?

Can health care providers order or demand HIV testing of patients for protection of such patients? Can health care providers who have experienced a potential exposure from a patient demand testing of the patient? Should all hospitalized patients be tested? Should all health care providers be tested?

There are other dimensions to the disclosure dilemma. Patients want information about health care providers who might have AIDS or be HIV positive, but health care providers also want to know which patients have been tested for HIV and which patients are positive for HIV. What responsibilities do employers such as hospitals and clinics have to advise patients of the HIV status of employees? What rights do HIV-positive health care providers have to privacy and to employment?

Judicial Council Opinion

It is important to respect patient autonomy and confidentiality as much as possible. Informed consent, specifically for HIV testing, must be obtained before testing. A patient may be tested without his or her consent if a health care provider is at risk for HIV infection because of contact with potentially infected bodily fluids. At risk patients should be encouraged to obtain testing.

Confidentiality may be waived when it is necessary to protect the public health or when necessary to protect individuals, including health care providers, who are endangered by persons infected with HIV. If an infected patient is endangering a third party, the physician should attempt to persuade the infected patient to cease endangering the third party. If that fails, the authorities should be notified. If they take no action, the physician should notify the endangered third party.

Denying treatment to an HIV-infected, HIV-seropositive patient, or to a patient who is unwilling to be tested is unethical except in a case in which knowledge of the patient's HIV status is vital to the patient's treatment. If a patient refuses after being informed of the physician's medical opinion, the physician would be justified in transferring care to another physician who is willing to abide by the patient's decision about testing.

LIFE AND DEATH DECISIONS

Quality of Life

Should every baby be saved? What if it is costing $2,000 per day to keep a two-pound baby alive? United States laws require doctors to begin treatment of all babies except those who would clearly not benefit. Unfortunately, no regulations guide a physician's decision to stop treatment. Limiting treatment to newborns is already common in Europe. Treatment begins immediately on all viable newborns in Britain, but the infant's status is reevaluated periodically, and if severe brain damage or death seems likely, efforts are stopped. This decision is made in Britain after consulting the parents; in France, it is made by a medical team.

Judicial Council Opinion

With regard to the treatment of severely deformed newborns and other people severely damaged by injury or illness, the quality of a person's life is one factor to consider in determining treatment.

The decision to treat a severely deformed newborn to the greatest extent possible belongs to the parents. The advice, knowledge, and cooperation of the physician should be readily available to the parents. They should be told their choices, expected benefits and risks, the infant's potential for social and intellectual development, and any other information that is relevant or desired.

Terminal Illness

The doctor is committed to prolonging life and relieving suffering. When these objectives conflict with each other, the doctor, patient, and/or family may resolve the conflict. With informed consent, the doctor may do what is medically necessary to alleviate severe pain or omit treatment in order to let a terminally ill patient die a natural death. However, a doctor should not intentionally cause death.

Patient Self-Determination Acts

The life-prolonging technology that has made the determination of death more difficult has also generated concern for many Americans. Adults of sound mind have the right to decide whether or not treatment will be received. They also have the right to determine whether life-prolonging technologies and machines will be used, and under what circumstances.

The lack of consistent laws coupled with inconsistent court decisions had left physicians and facilities without direction or defense. Individual states began working on solutions. Finally, the federal Patient Self-Determination Act became law in 1991.

All institutions, hospitals, hospices, HMOs, nursing facilities, and home care programs receiving funds from Medicare and Medicaid are required to give all adult patients written information about their right to accept or refuse medical and surgical treatment. They must also be given information about their right to formulate advance directives such as living wills and to designate someone to act on their behalf in making health care decisions using a durable power of attorney or medical proxy.

If a patient has prepared a living will, directive, or patient self-determination form, the doctor and office staff need to obtain a copy and document the patient's preferences.

The next step may be legislation regarding euthanasia; Washington and California have already had initiatives on the ballot. Washington Initiative 119 and California Proposition 161 failed to pass, but the concern and interest is apparent. The California proposition would have allowed mentally competent adults to instruct their doctors in writing to provide aid in dying upon their request when they become terminally ill. A person's decision to ask for aid in dying would be voluntary, and could be canceled at any time. The measure would have given the individual the option of having a doctor: (1) administer aid in dying; or (2) provide the means to the individual to self-administer aid in dying.

Determination of Death

The traditional way of determining death, and the one that is recognized as law in most states, is the irreversible cessation of heart, lung, and brain functions. However, technological advancements in recent years sometimes make possible continued functioning of the circulatory and respiratory systems through artificial support systems, even though all brain functions have irreversibly stopped. Because this is possible, most states have recognized—by statute or case law—that death can be determined on the basis of one factor alone: the permanent and irreversible loss of all brain functions.

Because state laws on the subject vary so much—in substance as well as language and style—several nationally recognized organizations have developed a model statute for the purpose of having it adopted in every state. The groups responsible for this model statute are the American Bar Association, the American Medical Association, the National Conference of Commissioners on Uniform State Laws, and the President's Commission for the Study of

Ethical Problems in Medicine and Biomedical Research. The proposed statute reads:

Uniform Determination of Death Act

An individual who has sustained either: (1) irreversible cessation of circulatory and respiratory functions, or (2) irreversible cessation of all functions of the entire brain, including the brain stem, is dead. A determination of death must be made in accordance with accepted medical standards.

The term "accepted medical standards" means that a doctor must use recognized and reliable tests and methods to determine the cessation and irreversibility of either cardiopulmonary or neurological functions.

PHYSICIAN RESPONSIBILITIES

Incompetent or Corrupt Practitioners

Judicial Council Opinion

A physician should never hesitate to expose, in an appropriate manner, incompetent, corrupt, dishonest, or unethical conduct by another member of the profession. Questions concerning a physician's conduct should first be brought before an appropriate medical committee or a committee appointed to deal with ethical relationships, assuming the delay in taking such a course would not impede the law. If the conduct is or might be unlawful, appropriate officers of the law should be promptly notified. Ethical physicians obey all laws concerning the practice of medicine and do not help others evade such laws.

COMPETENCY CHECK: SIX

12. True or false. Physicians are free to choose whom they will serve, but should respond to a request for assistance in an emergency.

13. True or false. A physician and staff need not obtain a copy of a patient's living will, health care power of attorney, or similar legal document.

SUMMARY

Ethics are those fundamental principles of right and wrong believed in by individuals and by groups of individuals—in this instance, medical and health care organizations.

In this chapter, we discussed the history of medical ethics as well as medical ethics today and the ethical standards of the medical and allied health professions as reflected in their organizations' codes of ethics.

Among the many areas touched on in these codes are financial issues, medical records, and relationships with others—including doctors and nonmedical personnel. Other areas of ethical concern are organ donation, allocation of scarce resources, fetal tissue research, abortion, genetic engineering, artificial insemination, determination of death, neglect of patients, terminal illness, and organ transplants.

Allied health professionals dedicate themselves to providing good quality health care with respect for human dignity, and pledge themselves to respect the law, to continue their education, to participate in community service, and to respect confidential patient information.

REFERENCES

1. *Current Opinion of the Judicial Council.* Chicago, Il: American Medical Association; 1981:15.

Appendix
Competency Check Answer Key

Chapter 1

COMPETENCY CHECK: ONE

1. True
2. True
3. True
4. False
5. a. Scientific advances that carry risks of undesirable results or side effects;
   b. Unrealistic expectations of a cure for every ailment;
   c. Poor communication between physician and patient;
   d. An increasingly litigious society.

COMPETENCY CHECK: TWO

6. Federal and state legislatures enact laws known as statutes (statutory law). Common laws are legal precedents established by judicial decisions.
7. Common law decisions are followed by other judges until the precedent is overruled by a court of higher authority. Common law may also be changed by statute.

8. Substantive law describes the rights and responsibilities of parties in legal relationships. Procedural law is concerned with how substantive law is implemented and how justice is administered.

COMPETENCY CHECK: THREE

9. True
10. True

Chapter 2

COMPETENCY CHECK: ONE

1. Medical Practice Act.
2. a. Fulfilling the prerequisite established by the state legislature and board of medical examiners.
   b. Reciprocity.
   c. Endorsement.

COMPETENCY CHECK: TWO

3. True
4. True

COMPETENCY CHECK: THREE

5. True
6. False

Chapter 3

1. a. The offer and acceptance.
   b. The consideration.
   c. The legal capacity to contract.
   d. Legal subject matter.
2. Legal capacity to contract means that the parties are mentally competent adults. Minors and those under legal disability do not have the legal capacity to contract.

3. This means that the physician must have and use reasonable skill, experience, and knowledge in treating the patients as would like physicians in the same circumstances.
4. a. Treating the patient as long as the patient's condition requires it or until a proper withdrawal or discharge is made.
   b. Informing patients of proposed treatment and obtaining appropriate consent before proceeding with treatment.
   c. Respecting the patient's privacy and confidential information acquired during the course of the physician-patient relationship.
5. He/she guarantees only that he/she has reasonable skill, experience and knowledge, and that he/she will exercise these attributes diligently in his/her treatment of the patient.
6. a. A patient is obligated to tell the physician the truth about the nature and duration of his/her symptoms and his/her medical history.
   b. The patient is expected to follow the physician's instructions completely.
   c. The patient is obligated to pay the physician for services rendered.

7. When a physician wishes to withdraw from a case, he/she must write the patient a letter, which is to be sent by certified mail with return receipt requested, containing the following elements:

   a. The statement that the physician is withdrawing and the reason why.
   b. The recommendation,

if appropriate, that the patient seek continued medical treatment. The physician should give the patient a reasonable amount of time (depending on the condition of the patient and his/her access to another physician) to do so before the effective termination date.

c. An offer to make information in the patient's medical records available to another physician only if the patient consents in writing to the release of the information.

d. The physician's signature. Copies of all communications should be filed with the patient's medical records.

8. The physician should send a letter confirming his/her dismissal to protect himself/herself in case it becomes necessary to prove that the physician did not abandon the patient but was discharged.

COMPETENCY CHECK: FOUR

9. Abandonment
10. Abandonment
11. The emancipated minor

12. The physician–patient relationship is limited to the treatment provided at the site of the emergency and is based on the victim's implied request for treatment.

Chapter 4

COMPETENCY CHECK: ONE

1. a. Specification of what data can be released.
    b. The name of the physician authorized to release information.
    c. The name of the intended recipient of the information.
    d. The date treatment was administered.
    e. The patient's signature, the date, and signature of a witness.

2. Patients may limit disclosure to treatment administered during a specified time for a certain condition. This patient should make sure the appropriate language is included in the disclosure authorization form.

COMPETENCY CHECK: TWO

3. True
4. True
5. a. Required by subpoena.
    b. Required by statute to

protect public health
and welfare.

c. Necessary for the
protection of the wel-
fare of the patient or
a third party.

6. a. Births and deaths.

b. Acts of violence,
such as gunshot
wounds and suspect-
ed cases of child
abuse.

c. Contagious, infec-
tious, or communica-
ble diseases.

COMPETENCY CHECK: THREE

7. By politely stating that
the matter will be referred
to the optometrist.

8. a. Appointment books,
patient records, and
other confidential
material should be
kept out of public
view.

b. There should be a
strictly enforced poli-
cy forbidding staff
from accessing
records to which they
are not privy.

c. Confidential discus-
sions with patients
should be private.

d. Patients and any facts
pertaining to them
should never be dis-
cussed outside the
office or in front of
other people inside
the office.

Chapter 5

COMPETENCY CHECK: ONE

1. True

2. The parent or legal
guardian of a minor child
must consent before the
minor receives any treat-
ment except in an emer-
gency; but, according to
the American Medical
Association, the minor's
consent should also be
obtained after the minor
reaches the age of 15.

COMPETENCY CHECK: TWO

3. To act for the benefit of
the patient. Included in
this obligation is the legal
duty to disclose voluntarily all information relevant
to the service or treatment
being performed.

4. The long-recognized principle that an adult of
"sound mind has the right
to determine what shall be
done to his/her body," and
the physician's obligation
to acquire a patient's consent before beginning
medical treatment.

5. a. The nature of the proposed treatment and
the effects it might
have on the patient's
body.

b. Normal risks and
hazards inherent in
the proposed treat-

ment and the likeli-
hood of each risk
occurring.
   c. Side effects or complications known nor-
mally to occur, their
severity, and perma-
nence.
   d. Alternative treatment,
including no treat-
ment, and the proba-
ble outcome of each.

COMPETENCY CHECK: THREE

6. Likelihood of occurrence,
severity, and permanence.
7. a. Consent is assumed,
as in any life- or
limb-threatening
emergency.
   b. The law requires a
certain treatment,
such as vaccinations
for school entry.
   c. A court order has
been issued, as might
occur if a parent
refuses lifesaving
treatment for a minor
child.
8. a. That the proposed
treatment is uncon-
ventional and experi-
mental.
   b. That all risks or side
effects may not be
known.
9. Occasionally, a condition
is discovered during
surgery that requires different or extended surgi-
cal treatment other than

that authorized by the
patient.

COMPETENCY CHECK: FOUR

10. Obtain proper authorization for the treatment,
thereby forcing the patient
to accept unwanted treat-
ment.
11. **Reasonable physician
standard:** The standard
of care provided by other
physicians in the same or
similar community, under
the same or similar cir-
cumstances.
**Reasonable person stan-
dard:** What another per-
son in the same or similar
circumstances would con-
sent to or allow.
12. A material risk is one that
a "reasonable person"
would consider signifi-
cant.

Chapter 6

COMPETENCY CHECK: ONE

1. A **tort** is a civil wrong
resulting from the breach
of a legal obligation for
which the court may pro-
vide a remedy.
2. **Negligence** is the failure
to meet the standard of
reasonable care.
3. **Professional negligence**
is the failure to meet the
"reasonable member of
the profession" standard.

An example would be the failure of a physician to see a patient often enough during the course of the patient's treatment to adequately monitor his/her condition.

4. The **standard of care** is that practiced by other doctors of similar training and standing, in the same or similar circumstances, and in the same or similar locale.

5. The locality rule was the legal principle that the standard of care in a negligence suit was that standard exercised or administered by physicians within the defendant's community. It was thought to be unfair to compare the standard of care practiced by a physician in a rural community with the standard of care practiced by a physician with access to a modern medical center. Today, even when the locality rule is applied, many courts no longer consider the prevailing community standard of paramount importance.

COMPETENCY CHECK: TWO

6. False
7. False
8. True
9. False

COMPETENCY CHECK: THREE

10. A judge or a jury of laypersons normally cannot be expected to know the standard of medical care, to determine whether it was met, or to identify the existence of proximate cause. The expert witness can define and explain these concepts.

11. An expert medical witness is one who, by virtue of his/her education and experience, has knowledge that the ordinary witness does not have. He/she may testify to known and assumed facts, give an opinion, and answer hypothetical questions.

12. The burden of proof automatically shifts to the defendant, who must prove a lack of negligence, or that negligence did not cause the patient's injury.

13. a. **Nominal damages:** Token compensation (usually one dollar) awarded when the court wishes to recognize that the plaintiff's legal rights were violated, although it has concluded that no actual loss was proved.

    b. **Actual or compen-**

satory damages:
Money awarded for
injuries or losses at-
tributable to the vio-
lation of the patient's
rights.

c. **Punitive damages:**
Compensation award-
ed beyond actual
damages as punish-
ment to the wrongdo-
er for the reckless
and malicious nature
of the wrongdoing.

COMPETENCY CHECK: FOUR

14. The doctrine of *respondeat superior* ("let the
master answer") is a rule
that holds the employer
responsible for the actions
of an employee or agent.
Liability of the employer
is limited to those acts
performed within the
scope of the employee's
or agent's responsibilities.
15. Physicians are liable for
the negligence of any
employee that occurs dur-
ing the course and in the
scope of the employee's
employment.
16. The physician can be
liable for any act of negligence by a hospital em-
ployee who is "borrowed"
by the physician to per-
form certain duties under
his/her direct supervision
and personal control.
17. An agency relationship

exists when, by mutual
consent:
a. One party (the agent)
agrees to work on
behalf of the other
(the principal); and
b. The agent's work is
subject to the control
of the principal.

Chapter 7

COMPETENCY CHECK: ONE

1. The change, who made it,
the date it was made, and
why it was made.
2. **Contributory negligence**
is a defense that claims
the conduct on the part of
the plaintiff (the patient)
contributed wholly or in
part to the harm or injury
allegedly caused by the
defendant.
3. Contributory negligence.
4. Damages are apportioned
according to the percent-
age of negligence by each
party.

COMPETENCY CHECK: TWO

5. The statutes of limitations
set a time on enforcement
of a right—the time peri-
od within which parties
must begin litigation. The
time limit varies accord-
ing to the type of case.
The purpose is to require
suits to be brought while
it is still possible to estab-

lish "reasonable standard
of care" as it pertains to
the case.
6. The day that the "reasonable person" discovers
negligence has occurred,
usually the date a second
physician identifies the
problem.
7. a. Fraudulent concealment by the physician
of the true nature of
the patient's condi-
tion.
b. The patient is
declared incompetent,
imprisoned, or other-
wise confined so that
he/she cannot pursue
his/her case.
c. A foreign object
being left in the body
during surgery.

Chapter 8

COMPETENCY CHECK: ONE

1. Assault and battery.
2. a. **Assault** is an intentional, deliberate
attempt, or threat to
attack or touch anoth-
er person without that
person's consent.
b. **Battery** is the touching of another person
without that person's
permission. In crimi-
nal law, the term
implies a forceful and
unlawful attack.

COMPETENCY CHECK: TWO

3. a. He was mentally
competent at the time
of detention.
b. That the commitment
was the result of mal-
ice, lack of good
faith, or failure to
comply with statutory
regulations.
4. If he voluntarily admits
his mistake, he may be
liable to a charge of negligence, an unintentional
tort. If he does not dis-
close the error, he may be
liable for fraud, an intentional tort.

COMPETENCY CHECK: THREE

5. False
6. True

COMPETENCY CHECK: FOUR

7. The medical assistant
should seek legal advice,
since he/she may have to
later prove that undue
influence was not applied.

COMPETENCY CHECK: FIVE

8. Murder is unlawful killing
that is willful and deliberate. Manslaughter is the
unlawful killing of a
human being with no mal-
ice or intent to kill.
9. a. Acts classified as
criminal offenses
must be specifically

established and carefully defined by state or federal statute. Offenses classified as **torts** are only generally defined in statutory law and are usually subject to judicial interpretation.

b. **Crimes** are considered offenses against the state and/ or public welfare. **Torts** are wrongs against individuals.

c. In **criminal cases**, the defendant must be proven "guilty beyond a shadow of a doubt." In **civil (tort) cases**, the plaintiff must prove his/her case by a "preponderance of evidence."

COMPETENCY CHECK: SIX

10. True
11. True
12. True
13. False
14. True
15. True

Chapter 9

COMPETENCY CHECK: ONE

1. A body cannot be disposed of until the physician has completed the medical portion of a death certificate, signed it and transmitted it to the funeral director in charge of funeral arrangements.

2. a. The cause is unknown.
   b. The deceased was not attended by a physician at the time of death or for a reasonable amount of time preceding the death.
   c. The attending physician was unable to establish a diagnosis before the patient died.

3. To protect the general health and well-being of their populations.

4. True

COMPETENCY CHECK: TWO

5. To prevent people who are illegally using drugs from obtaining drugs. It creates a closed system of distribution—a system accessible only to legitimate handlers.

6. **Schedule II.** These drugs have a high potential for abuse even though they have accepted medicinal uses.

COMPETENCY CHECK: THREE

7. a. The full name and address of the patient for whom the drug was intended.
   b. The date the drug

was given or pre-
scribed.

c. The quantity and
character of the drug
and how it was dis-
pensed. Dispensing
records must be kept
for two years.

8. The Drug Enforcement
Administration.

9. a. The physician's bag
should be stored in
the office in a place
inaccessible to
patients. If it must be
left in a car, it should
be locked in the
trunk.

b. Prescription pads
should be kept under
lock and key except
for the single pad
currently in use.

c. Prescription pads
should be designed
and printed to mini-
mize the possibility
of alteration.

Chapter 10

COMPETENCY CHECK: ONE

1. False
2. True
3. False
4. False

COMPETENCY CHECK: TWO

5. The assistant should tactfully, but firmly, insist
that the friend wait in the
waiting room.

6. A single line should be
drawn through the incor-
rect data and a note
should be made in the
margin indicating who
made the change, when,
and why. The correct data
should then be entered in
chronological order on the
correct chart.

7. The results of a test or
procedure are crucial to a
patient's legal claim; the
omitted information may
suggest negligence or
carelessness. The entry
will clearly indicate that
the test or procedure was
performed, even if the
results were normal.

COMPETENCY CHECK: THREE

8. The fact that the patient
has not paid his bill does
not affect his right to have
his records transferred to
another physician.

9. His/her prime objective is
to protect and preserve
the integrity of the sub-
poenaed records.

10. An official receipt for the
records.

11. The custodian of the
records may have to sign
a sworn statement that the
photocopy is a faithful
reproduction of the original record. Or, he/she may
have to take both the original and the photocopy to

court, where a court-appointed officer will compare the two documents to make sure the copy is an exact duplicate.

Chapter 11

1. To provide, without regard to fault, medical care and compensation for the injured employee and his/her dependents; to provide rehabilitation if necessary; to encourage the employer's interest in safety; and to promote safety in the workplace.
2. OSHA legislation was passed in an attempt to ensure that employees are provided with a workplace that is free from recognized hazards that cause serious injury or death.
3. Employees must comply with OSHA standards, follow employer safety and health rules, use protective equipment and clothing when necessary, and report hazardous conditions.
4. **Right-to-know regulations** give the health care employee and others the right to information about toxic hazards and the protective equipment to use when handling such mate-

rials. A **MSDS** is a Material Safety Data Sheet. It lists each ingredient in a product.

5. According to regulations, health care offices must have:
   a. a list of all employees who might be exposed to blood-borne diseases on either a regular or an occasional basis.
   b. a written exposure control plan.
   c. one employee in charge of OSHA compliance.
   d. availability of protective equipment and clothing.
   e. an employee training program in writing, and records of sessions and participants.
   f. warning labels and signs denoting biohazards.
   g. written guidelines for identifying, containing, and disposing of medical waste in accordance with state and local laws; the method for housecleaning and decontamination, including laundry.
   h. written guidelines for

procedures to follow if an employee is exposed to blood or other potentially infectious materials, as well as a policy for reporting incidents of exposure and maintaining records.

   i. postexposure evaluation procedures.

6. Body fluids include semen, blood, vaginal secretions, synovial fluid, pleural fluid, pericardial fluid, cerebrospinal fluid, amniotic fluids, and saliva.

7. True

8. False. Infectious wastes may be incinerated by the facility, or must be placed in special puncture-resistant or lead-lined containers and removed by a medical waste disposal company.

COMPETENCY CHECK: THREE

9. True

10. False. Overtime is considered any work exceeding 40 hours per week; time off may not be given in lieu of pay.

11. Yes, the employer is required to pay overtime.

12. The Social Security Act provides retirement benefits, disability benefits, dependent benefits, survivor benefits, and Medicare.

COMPETENCY CHECK: FOUR

13. Some state and local statutes prohibit discrimination on the basis of sexual orientation, personal appearance, mental health, mental retardation, marital status, parenthood, and political affiliation.

14. In the 1970s, the Equal Employment Opportunity Commission defined sexual harassment as unwelcome sexual advances or requests for sexual favors. In the 1980s, the EEOC broadened the definition to include other verbal or physical conduct of a sexual nature when: (1) submission to such conduct is made either explicitly or implicitly a term or condition of an individual's employment; (2) submission to or rejection of such conduct by an individual is used as a basis for employment decisions affecting such individual; or (3) such conduct has the purpose or effect of unreasonably interfering with an individual's work performance or creating an intimidating, hostile, or offensive work environment.

15. True

16. False. This statute applies to individuals with substantial (as distinct from minor) impairments. These must be impairments that limit major life activities. The law does not apply to individuals with minor nonchronic conditions of short duration, such as a broken arm or leg.
17. True
18. True
19. True

COMPETENCY CHECK: SIX

20. Unpaid leave must be granted for any of the following reasons:
    a. to care for the employee's child after birth, adoption, or foster care placement; or
    b. to care for the employee's spouse, son or daughter, or parent who has a serious health condition; or
    c. for a serious health condition that makes the employee unable to perform his/her job.
21. Federal and state laws require covered employers to provide up to twelve weeks per year of unpaid, job-protected leave to eligible employees for certain family and medical reasons.
22. For the duration of the leave, the employer must maintain the employee's coverage under any group health plan. Upon return from the leave, most employees must be restored to their original or equivalent positions with equivalent pay, benefits, and other employment terms. The use of the leave cannot result in the loss of any employment benefit that accrued prior to the start of the employee's leave.

Chapter 12

COMPETENCY CHECK: ONE

1. True
2. False. Financial information about patients is as confidential as the health care information. Interviews regarding financial matters need to be conducted in private.

COMPETENCY CHECK: TWO

3. Age, marital status, sex, color, race, national origin, receipt of public assistance, or exercising rights under consumer credit laws.

4. False
5. If the patient is informed in advance, fees for multiple or complex insurance forms, interest or finance charges, and fees for missed appointments that have not been canceled within a specific time.
6. False. The statute of frauds requires certain contracts to be in writing.
7. False
8. A truth in lending statement must be completed if there will be more than four payments and there is a bilateral agreement.

COMPETENCY CHECK: THREE

9. True
10. Collection practices that are illegal are: (1) threatening action that will not be taken; (2) use of abusive or vulgar language; (3) using deceptive or unfair methods; (4) contacting the debtor more than once a week.

COMPETENCY CHECK: FOUR

11. The lien ensures that the doctor or facility is paid from any sums received by any settlement or compromise that the patient may obtain from the adverse party.
12. The two basic purposes of the federal bankruptcy

laws are: (1) to provide relief and protection to debtors who have become insolvent; and (2) to provide a fair method of distributing a debtor's assets among all creditors.

Chapter 13

COMPETENCY CHECK: ONE

1. a. The first phase of a suit is called the pleadings phase. This phase consists primarily of three legal documents designed to identify the controversial or disputed issues to be decided during trial: the complaint, the answer, and the reply.
   b. The second phase is called the pretrial discovery period. The main purpose of this period is to permit the parties to uncover all relevant information before the trial.
   c. The trial phase is next. The purpose of the trial is to hear the case in a neutral environment and to achieve a just settlement of the dispute.
   d. An appeal can be filed if there is evidence that suggests the strong possibility

of error, injustice, or impropriety during the trial court proceedings. The appeal must be based on an issue of law, rather than on the jury's decision concerning a fact or facts.

2. The correct sequence is complaint, answer, depositions, jury selection, opening statements, evidence of plaintiff, evidence of defendant, closing statements of the plaintiff and defendant, verdict, judgment, and appeal.

COMPETENCY CHECK: TWO

3. a. To eliminate claims with no merit.
   b. To help plaintiffs with legitimate claims to obtain expert witnesses.

4. a. Preclaim agreements: The provider of a health care service and the patient agree before a service is rendered that if a dispute arises concerning the service it will be settled through arbitration rather than litigation.
   b. Postclaim agreements are executed after a dispute arises; both sides agree to have it resolved through arbitration rather than litigation.

5. Any three of the following:
   a. Cases are solved more quickly than they are in the courtroom, thereby saving litigants time, money, and aggravation.
   b. The panelists are usually more knowledgeable about technical medical matters than is the typical juror or judge.
   c. There is less publicity, and therefore less damage to a physician's reputation.
   d. The atmosphere and rules regarding admissibility and relevancy of evidence are more relaxed than those enforced during a trial.
   e. There is some evidence that arbitration panels are less likely to make excessive, emotionally-induced awards than are juries or judges.

COMPETENCY CHECK: THREE

6. The purpose of QA/RM is to provide quality patient care.

7. Some common issues for risk management are ap-

pointment delays, insensi-
tivity to patient concerns,
unsafe facilities, injection
or minor surgery errors,
specimen collection and
labeling errors, improper
procedures for infection
control, and lack of documentation of quality con-
trol in laboratories (e.g.
calibration of equipment).
8. False
9. The six basic guidelines
   for health care practitioners are:
   a. Always demonstrate
      a feeling of genuine
      concern for the wel-
      fare of all patients.
   b. Always respect the
      confidentiality of the
      patient–doctor rela-
      tionship.
   c. Never go beyond the
      scope and training of
      your field.
   d. Always obey federal
      and state laws as well
      as local ordinances.
   e. Conscientiously fol-
      low the procedures
      designed to provide
      the best of care and
      facilitate understand-
      ing between health
      care provider and
      patient.
   f. Keep current on the
      changes in your field
      and in the health care
      field in general.

Chapter 14

COMPETENCY CHECK: ONE

1. False
2. True
3. False

COMPETENCY CHECK: TWO

4. The patient's attorney and
   the patient's insurance
   company.

COMPETENCY CHECK: THREE

5. True
6. False

COMPETENCY CHECK: FOUR

7. False
8. True

COMPETENCY CHECK: FIVE

9. False
10. False
11. True

COMPETENCY CHECK: SIX

12. True
13. False

Glossary

A

Abandonment: The voluntary relinquishment of right, title, or claim with the intention of not reclaiming or not repossessing that being given up. With regard to the physician–patient relationship, abandonment is conduct that is positively and unequivocally inconsistent with the nature of the contract, such as the improper severance of the physician–patient relationship.

Acceptance: The voluntary consent to terms of an offer.

Accessory: One who helps another commit a crime in a secondary way or as a subordinate.

Accessory after-the-fact: One who assists a felon knowing the felon is being sought for the commission or attempted commission of a crime in order to help the felon escape punishment.

Accessory before-the-fact: One who orders or assists in the commission of a crime, but is not present during its perpetration.

Accomplice: One who voluntarily and knowingly and with common intent participates with another in the commission or attempted commission of a crime and who is liable for the identical offense as is the other offender.

Acquit: To set free or absolve an individual of an accusation or charge of guilt. An acquittal occurs at the end of a trial when a judge or jury decides that the defendant is not guilty of the charges levied against him.

Action: The legal and formal demand of one's right from another party made in a court of law.

Actionable: A wrongdoing that may form the basis of civil cause of action.

Ad hoc (for this; for this particular purpose): An ad hoc committee is one formed for a particular purpose. The committee is dissolved once its purpose is fulfilled.

Admission: A statement by the accused (usually the defendant) that tends to support the charge against him/her; the voluntary acknowledgment or confession of certain facts that tend to support the adversary position.

Request for admissions: Pretrial discovery tool whereby one party asks the other to admit or deny certain admissions.

Adversary: An opponent in a legal controversy.

Adversary process or system: The positioning of opposing sides against each other, giving each side the opportunity to prove or disprove disputed issues in a fair and legally prescribed manner.

Adverse party: The opposing litigant in a suit or legal action.

Affidavit: A voluntary, written statement made under oath before an officer of the court or before a notary public.

Affirm: To confirm, establish, reassert; also, an appellate court ruling that the judgment or decision of a lower court is correct and should stand.

Affirmative defense: The presentation of new evidence by defense to show that plaintiff's complaints are attributable to some cause other than defendant's negligence.

Agent: A person authorized by another person to act for him/her, usually in business matters; one who acts for another on the basis of mutual consent.

Alien: An individual who is not a citizen of the country.

Allegation: An assertion of fact; a statement of what a litigant expects to prove.

Allege: To assert, state, or charge certain facts.

Amicus curiae **(friend of the court):** One who calls the court's attention to a matter that could otherwise be missed or one who offers the court information on a legal point in a brief.

Answer: A defendant's formal written response to plaintiff's complaint in which defendant's grounds for a defense are stated. The answer is submitted during the pleadings phase of the litigation. It is known in some jurisdictions as the "plea."

Appeal: To petition a superior court to review and correct a decision and an alleged error made by a lower court.

Appellant: Party appealing decision by a lower court.

Appellate court: A court having the authority to review the law applied to a case in a lower court. This court, which reviews only issues of law, has authority to affirm, modify, set aside, or reverse earlier decisions.

Appellee: Party in an action who does not want an appellate court to set aside or modify the decision made in a lower court.

Arbitration: A process whereby a dispute is settled by impartial individual(s) appointed by mutual consent of the parties or by statutory authority.

Arbitrator: A disinterested private person chosen by the parties in a dispute to decide a controversy.

Artifice: Subtle deception, which is often a fraudulent device; usually implies intent to trick or deceive.

Assault: An intentional, deliberate attempt, or threat to, inflict bodily harm on another person; to threaten to attack or touch another without consent.

Attest: To affirm as true; to corroborate; to sign one's name as witness to the execution of a document.

Autopsy: The physical and/or microscopic examination of a dead body and its parts to determine cause of death.

B

Bankrupt: A party that is unable to pay its debts.

Bankruptcy: The state of being bankrupt as so ordered by a court of law.

Battery: The touching of another person without permission. In criminal law, the term implies a forceful and unlawful attack. When a physician provides treatment in excess of what a patient consents to, the physician commits a technical battery for which the patient may seek legal redress.

Bench: Refers to the court, to the judges collectively, or to the place where a trial judge sits.

Bench trial: A trial held before a judge without a jury; a jury-waived trial.

Bind: To place under legal obligation by contract or oath. Example: The Oath of Hippocrates binds physicians to keep information regarding their patients confidential.

Board of Medical Examiners: A state administrative agency empowered to examine the qualifications of applicants for medical licenses and to issue licenses to qualified applicants.

Borrowed servant doctrine: A legal theory in which a person (the "servant") employed by one entity is "borrowed" by another to perform certain duties under the borrower's direct supervision and total control. Under such circumstances, the borrower rather than the employer may be liable for the employee's negligence.

Breach: Failure to perform a legal obligation by commission or omission.

Breach of contract: Failure to meet a contractual obligation without legal excuse.

Breach of duty: Not performing, or performing incorrectly, an obligation to an individual or to society.

Brief: A written document, prepared by an attorney on behalf of a client and submitted to court, that cites arguments and authorities supporting the client's position on certain matters.

Burden of proof: The responsibility of proving the facts in a disputed issue; the responsibility of plaintiff except in cases based on *res ipsa loquitur.*

C

Case: An action or cause for action; a matter in dispute; a suit.

Cause of action: Set of facts that gives someone the right to seek legal redress.

Caveat emptor **(let the buyer beware):** Expresses the principle that the purchaser buys at his/her own risk.

Certification: A process in most medical and allied health occupations through which practitioners exhibit competence or merit by voluntarily participating in evaluation programs meant to measure some degree of knowledge, ability, or skill. Those who meet stipulated criteria are awarded certification.

Chain of custody of specimens: Proof establishing the sequence of possession of a specimen that is offered into evidence in a legal situation.

Civil: Pertaining to legal rights between private individuals and to legal proceedings concerning those rights.

Civil action: Legal action taken to protect or enforce a private right or to remedy a wrongdoing.

Civil law: That branch of law governing the rights of individuals as private citizens; a branch of law generally concerned with noncriminal matters.

Code: Statutes enacted by live bodies and published in volumes, usually according to subject matter (e.g., the motor vehicle code, the penal code); a body of laws pertaining to one subject.

Coercion: The act of compelling someone by threat, force, or arms to act against his/her will.

Common law: That body of law based on judicial precedents or usage and custom rather than on statutes. Sometimes called case law.

Comparative negligence: A doctrine that seeks to apportion damages between two litigants, both of whom were negligent to some degree, according to the percentage of damage each litigant caused. In practice, damages awarded plaintiff are reduced by the percentage of damage attributable to plaintiff's own negligence.

Complaint: A legal document stating the plaintiff's cause of action and the grounds on which the defendant is being sued; the first pleading by the plaintiff in a civil action. Known in some jurisdictions as the declaration.

Consideration: The contractual element through which something of value is given or promised in exchange for something or the promise of something; often the mutual exchange of promises, such as the patient promised to pay a surgeon who promises to perform an operation. The consideration distinguishes a contract from a gift.

Contempt of court: A term covering open disrespect and/or willful disobedience of a court order; conduct that hinders the administration of justice.

Contingency fee: A fee arrangement between attorney and client that hinges upon the successful resolution of a civil case. In civil negligence cases, it is often an agreed-upon or regulated percentage of the party's monetary recovery. Contingency fees for handling criminal cases are considered unethical.

Contract: An agreement involving two or more competent parties in which each is obligated to the other to fulfill promises made. The law provides a remedy if one party fails to meets its obligation as established in the contract.

Express contract: A contract in which the terms are explicit and clearly stated, orally or in writing. Some contracts must be written to be enforceable.

Implied contract: A contract that can be inferred by reasonable people from the actions and conduct of the parties.

Contributory negligence: A defense in which the defendant claims that the plaintiff's negligence is wholly or partially responsible for the harm allegedly caused by the defendant. When presented as an affirmative defense in a medical negligence case, the defendant–physician must prove that the plaintiff failed to act as a reasonable patient would have acted in the same circumstances.

Controlled substances: Narcotics and other dangerous drugs whose manufacture, distribution, and dispensing is controlled by the federal government.

Coroner: A public official who investigates any death not attributable to natural causes.

Counterclaim: A demand by the defendant that opposes a demand by a plaintiff; a cause of action asserted by the defendant.

Course and scope of employment: A term referring to those duties an employee is hired and expected to perform while engaged in the service of the employer.

Court: That part of the judicial branch of government whose function is to apply laws to disputes brought before it and to administer justice.

Court order: Instructions by the court (usually a judge) to do something pertaining to the case being heard.

Crime: An act clearly identified and defined by statute as a wrong against public welfare, for which the offender will be prosecuted by the state or federal government.

Cross-examination: The questioning of a witness by the opposing counsel who often attempts to discredit or confuse the witness in the testimony.

D

Damages: Monetary compensation awarded by law to one who has suffered loss, detriment, or injury to his/her person, property, or rights because of another's negligence or other wrongful act.

Nominal damages: A token or trivial amount, often $1 awarded to recognize the violation of a right when no actual harm, suffering, or loss was proved by the plaintiff.

Compensatory damages: An award for the monetary value of actual losses sustained, such as medical expenses, loss of wages, etc.

Punitive damages: An award in excess of the plaintiff's actual losses which is made to punish the wrongdoer for misconduct judged by the court to be malicious or willful. Punitive damages are also known as exemplary damages.

DEA (Drug Enforcement Administration): The federal agency within the Justice Department responsible for enforcing provisions of the Comprehensive Drug Abuse Prevention and Control Act of 1970 (The Controlled Substances Act).

Deadly weapon: Any instrument capable of causing death or serious bodily harm; some instruments are inherently deadly, such as guns or knives; others are deadly on the basis of how they are used—e.g., wrenches or hammers.

Decedent: One who has ceased living; a deceased person.

Declaration: See Complaint.

Defamation of character: The damaging of a person's character, name, or reputation by false and malicious statements. A written false and malicious statement constitutes libel. An oral malicious statement constitutes slander.

Default: Not performing an obligation to one's own disadvantage; in the context of judicial proceedings, the failure to take necessary procedural steps thereby resulting in judgment against the person defaulting.

Defendant: Person against whom legal action is taken; in civil suits, the person being sued; in criminal action, the person being prosecuted.

Defense: The denial, response, or plea opposing the truth of the plaintiff's allegations against the defendant; that put forward by defendant to diminish plaintiff's case.

Demurrer: Formal allegation by defendant that even if the facts stated in the plaintiff's complaint are true, they are not legally sufficient to constitute a just cause of action.

Denial defense: To refute or contradict the allegation made by plaintiff.

Deposition: A method of uncovering evidence in which one party questions the other party or a witness for the other party before the trial. This is done in the presence of a court reporter who records, verbatim, the questions and answers, which are given under oath. A transcript is made of the proceedings and often submitted as evidence during the trial.

Directed verdict: A decision returned by the jury solely on the basis of the judge's instructions. The judge may instruct the jury to find for either party if the opposing side fails to present an adequate case or defense.

Dismissal: A denial; a cancellation. To dismiss a motion is to deny it; to dismiss an appeal is to place the parties in the same position as though no appeal had been submitted—in other words, to affirm the judgment of the lower court.

District court: A trial court with territorial jurisdiction over certain cases that arise within the boundaries of its territory. U.S. District Courts have jurisdiction over offenses involving federal laws and suits involving litigants from different states.

Docket: An official record containing brief entries describing certain acts performed in connection with a case; also the name given to the list of cases to be tried by a court.

Donee: The recipient of a gift.

Doctrine: A rule, theory, principle, or set of principles.

Domestic violence: Violence involving individuals who are related by blood or marriage or are sharing a dwelling or home in a nontraditional family-type relationship.

Donor: One who makes a gift.

Due care: The amount or standard of care required; reasonable care; that degree of care a reasonable person or a reasonable member of a profession would exercise under the same or similar circumstances.

Due process of law: A phrase used to convey the principle that fair procedures must be used whenever the freedom, property, and/or rights of an individual are to be abridged, restricted, or rescinded by governmental actions. Fair procedures include giving the accused in a criminal matter written notice of the charges against him/her and permitting the accused the opportunity to be heard and to present a defense.

Duress: The act of compelling another by force or threat to do something the person does not want to do.

Duty: A legal or moral obligation.

E

Emancipated minor: Someone under the age of majority who lives independently of his/her parents and is entirely self-supporting. An emancipated minor is responsible for his/her own debts, and may enter into contracts.

Embezzlement: The unlawful taking of the property of another by a party entrusted with the property.

Estate: The interest in property of an individual.

Euthanasia: The act of causing the death of a terminally ill individual; mercy killing.

Ethics: A moral code; the standards of behavior members of certain groups agree to uphold and to be governed by.

Expert witness: See Witness.

Express contract: See Contract.

F

False imprisonment: The unlawful restraint of another's personal liberty; coercion that prevents another person from exercising his/her powers of locomotion.

Federal courts: Courts of the United States established under the U. S. Constitution or by the U. S. Congress.

Federal Tort Claims Act: A federal law enacted in 1946 that partially abolished the federal government's immunity from tort liability by granting private individuals the right to sue the U.S. government for losses and injuries suffered because of negligence by a government employee.

Felony: A term used to distinguish more serious crimes from less serious crimes, which are known as misdemeanors. Many statutes define a felony as an offense for which the punishment is one or more years of imprisonment or death.

Fiduciary: A provider of certain services who is obligated to act in the best interest of the person being served.

Fiduciary relationship: A relationship in which the provider of services must act in the best interest of the person being served. Examples: physician–patient, attorney–client, and priest–parishioner.

Fraud: A misrepresentation made with the intent to deceive. The misrepresentation can be concealment or nondisclosure of certain important information, as well as false representations.

G

Garnishment: The process pursuant to statute under which property is attached in order to obtain payment of a debt; the property of a judgment debtor that is held by a third party.

Good faith: The honest and sincere intent to fulfill one's obligations; the total lack of desire to seek or obtain unfair advantage over another.

Good Samaritan law: A statute enacted in most states that grants immunity for ordinary negligence to individuals who provide first aid at the site of accidents.

Grand jury: See Jury.

Gross negligence: See Negligence.

H

Harassment: The state of being troubled, harried, worried, or tormented by repeated attacks.

Hearing: A proceeding before a judge in which evidence is submitted in order to try an issue of fact and to reach a decision. Generally, a hearing is less formal than a trial.

Hearsay evidence: Testimony based on what a witness heard someone else say, not what the witness himself/herself saw, knows, or dealt with personally.

Hung jury: One that cannot reconcile its members' differences of opinion and, therefore, cannot reach a decision.

I

Immune: Exempt or free from duty or penalty; not subject to liability.

Immoral conduct: Behavior that falls below standards of conduct subscribed to by respectable members of a group or community.

Implied contract: See Contract.

Incompetency: The inability—for physical, intellectual, or moral reasons—to conduct one's affairs. An incompetent person cannot enter into contracts.

Independent contractor: A person who agrees to do certain work but retains control over how the work gets done.

Informed consent: An agreement to allow something to be done based on a complete explanation of the procedure, material risks inherent therein, and alternatives.

Injunction: A court order prohibiting someone from a specific action.

Instructions (to the jury): The judge's statement to the jury before the jury begins its deliberations made for the purpose of advising the jury on the law applicable to the case.

Interrogatory: A method of pretrial discovery in which a written set of questions is served by one party on its adversary, who must reply in writing under oath.

Intestate: To die without leaving a valid will.

Invasion of privacy: The violation of one's right to be left alone and to live without being subject to unwarranted or undesired publicity.

Issue: A matter disputed between two parties. The dispute may be of fact or law.

J

Joint screening panel: A group of people, usually physicians and attorneys, which is organized to review legal claims against physicians and to determine if there is merit to any claim.

Judge: The head of a court who presides at all sessions, resolves disputes of legal issues, and resolves disputes of factual issues in the absence of a jury. Sometimes called a jurist.

Judgment: The final decision of a court regarding the rights and claims of parties involved in litigation.

Judgment by default: A decision in favor of one party, made because the other party failed to appear in court at the specified time.

Judgment notwithstanding the verdict: A judgment by the court, despite an opposite verdict reached by the jury.

Jurisdiction: The authority of a court to try a case. It must cover subject matter as well as territory.

Jurisprudence: The philosophy of law; the study of law and its legal systems.

Jury: A panel of men and women sworn to decide issues of fact at a trial.

>*Grand jury:* A group of people, usually 23, that investigates crimes committed within a certain jurisdiction and indicts people for crimes when it believes there is sufficient evidence to hold a trial.

>*Petit jury:* The ordinary trial jury, usually composed of 12 members.

Justice: The goal of rendering every person his/her due according to principles of fairness; the administration of law. A title given to judges, particularly judges of U.S. and state supreme courts and of some appellate courts.

L

Law: Those rules and principles of conduct required of citizens by legislative enactments or court decisions.

Legacy: Money or property bequeathed by will.

Liable: Responsible for; legally obligated.

Liability: A legal obligation to do or not to do something.

Libel: False and malicious written statement(s) made to defame a person's character, name, or reputation.

License: A permit granted by a governmental agency giving the recipient permission to do something he/she could not do without the license.

Lien: A claim on the property of another as security for a debt.

Litigant: A party involved in a lawsuit—defendant or plaintiff.

Litigation: Civil controversy contested in a court; lawsuit.

Living will: A legal instrument which states that the individual signing it desires not to be kept alive by life support measures in the event of a terminal illness or injury.

Locality rule: The practice of using the standard of a local community as the standard against which a person's conduct is measured.

M

Majority, age of: The age at which a person is legally responsible for his/her own actions, including contracts and debts, and is entitled to certain civic rights. Traditionally, the age was 21, but in most states the age has been lowered to 18.

Malfeasance: The doing of an unlawful act.

Misfeasance: The improper performance of a lawful act.

Malice: The intent, without justification or excuse, to commit an act that will cause injury or harm to another person or persons.

Manslaughter: The unlawful killing of someone without malice or intent. Gross negligence which causes the death of a person may subject the offender to a charge of involuntary manslaughter.

Material risk: A risk that a reasonable person would consider important, significant, and necessary to know; a risk that a person should be informed of before asked to consent to a procedure in which the risk might occur.

Medical examiner: A physician, often a pathologist, who is publicly charged with the responsibility of investigating sudden, unexplained, and unnatural deaths. This responsibility includes the performance of autopsies to determine the cause of death.

Medical practice act: A state statute governing the practice of medicine in that state.

Mens rea **(a guilty mind):** The mental state accompanying the doing of an illegal act.

Merits: The substance of a litigant's claim or defense.

Minor: A person under the age of majority.

Misdemeanor: A class of criminal offenses less serious than felonies, one for which the penalties are less severe.

Mistrial: A trial declared void before a verdict is rendered.

Moral turpitude: Outrageous vileness, baseness, or dishonesty.

Motion: A formal request that the court or judge make an order or ruling in the applicant's favor.

N

Negligence: Failure to meet the standards of reasonable care; not using care a reasonable person would have used in doing something, or not doing something a reasonable person would have done.

> *Gross negligence:* Failure to use even slight care in the performance of duty; wanton, reckless disregard for the welfare of another.

> *Negligence per se:* Behavior that can be declared negligent without proof or argument because it violates a law or is an obvious disregard of prudence.

***Non compos mentis* (not having control over the mind or intellect):** A general term covering all forms of insanity.

Nonfeasance: Failure to do something that should have been done.

Nonsuit: A decision against the plaintiff when he/she is unable to prove a case or when he/she does not proceed to trial. The decision is not based on the merits of the case and, therefore, does not prevent another action.

Notary public: A public officer with authority to administer oaths, attest documents, and take depositions; may also be a private individual who applies for and receives authority to act as a notary in the witnessing of documents.

O

Oath: A declaration to tell the truth, an affirmation that what has been told is the truth, or a declaration to perform in a faithful and truthful manner.

Offer: That element of a contract indicating an interest in or willingness to establish a contract. With regard to the physician–patient contract, the offer is usually the patient's request for treatment.

Opinion: The explanation behind a court's judgment; the reason for the judgment.

Ordinance: A local law or rule; the rules adopted by a municipality.

Ordinary negligence: See Negligence.

P

Perjury: The criminal offense of making of false statements under oath.

Petition: The equivalent of a complaint. See Complaint.

Plaintiff: A person who, feeling wronged, initiates a lawsuit to remedy the wrong.

Pleadings: The first phase of a lawsuit during which the issues in dispute are identified and clarified, including the plaintiff's cause of action and the defendant's grounds of defense.

***Post mortem* (after death):** See Autopsy.

Power of attorney: A written document stating that one person, the principal, has given another person, the agent, authority to act in certain matters on behalf of the principal.

Precedent: A court decision that establishes a legal principle on which subsequent similar cases are tried and decided; a previously decided case recognized as authority for deciding subsequent cases.

Preponderance of evidence: Evidence that is more convincing than evidence entered in opposition; evidence of greater weight or credibility .

Pretrial discovery: The phase of litigation during which both parties accumulate evidence to support their positions and during which the issues are further clarified.

***Prima facie* (at first view):** A fact presumed to be true in the absence of contrary evidence.

Principal: The person, with regard to the law of agency, who permits or directs another to act for the benefit of the principal and who is subject to the principal's control.

Private law: The branch of law governing certain activities between and among private individuals; sometimes called civil law.

Privileged communications: Communications between and among certain parties that are protected, by law, from forced disclosure in a court of law. Attorney–client, physician–patient, and husband–wife communications are usually privileged.

Probate: The process of establishing the validity of a will in court.

Probate court: A court that deals exclusively with matters of probate and of administering estates.

Procedural law: The category of law dealing with the mechanics and methods of the legal process; the rules and practices through which justice is administered.

Proof: Evidence that leads to the establishment of a fact in the mind of a judge or juror.

Prosecution: The process of pursuing a lawsuit or criminal trial; the party initiating a criminal trial; the state.

Prosecutor: A public official responsible for seeing that laws are executed and enforced. Usual duties are to investigate and pursue prosecution of people accused of crimes.

Proximate cause: An action or inaction that, in a natural, direct, continuous, and unbroken sequence, produces an injury that would not have occurred otherwise.

Public law: The branch of law defining and governing rights and responsibilities between government and citizens.

Q

***Qui facit per alium facit per se* (he who acts through another acts himself):** The doctrine that acts of an agent are the acts of the principal.

R

Reasonable person: A term that refers to a hypothetical person who possesses and exercises the attention, knowledge, intelligence, and judgment that society expects and requires all citizens to possess and exercise in order to protect their own interests and the interests of others; also known as a reasonably prudent person or an ordinarily prudent man.

Rebut: To refute; to present opposing evidence or arguments.

Recovery: The judgment of a court establishing the right of a litigant to "recover" or get back that which was lost. The term is often used with regard to the amount of the judgment.

Redress: Action taken to rectify, correct, or remedy a wrong. Satisfaction for damages incurred.

Release: The relinquishment of a right, title, or claim to someone else; often used in reference to the document setting forth the relinquishment.

Remand: Send back. An appellate court sometimes has a case remanded, or sent back to the court from which it came for further action.

Remedy: The way of redressing or compensating for an injury; usually a monetary award.

Reply: A pleading by the plaintiff that answers a new issue raised in the defendant's answer, such as an affirmative defense or counterclaim.

Res ipsa loquitur **(the thing speaks for itself):** A doctrine whereby the negligence of the alleged wrongdoer (defendant) may be inferred because of the existence of certain facts.

Res judicata **(the thing has been decided):** Refers to the rule that once a matter has been tried and decided, the decision is final and the matter cannot be retried on the same evidence.

Rescind: To negate, void, or nullify an agreement or contract whereby the parties are restored to the position held before the agreement or contract was established.

Respondeat superior **(let the master answer):** A rule that holds the master/employer/or principal responsible for the negligence of a servant/employee/or agent. Liability of an employer or principal is limited to those acts performed within the course and scope of the employee's or agent's responsibility.

Review: A judicial examination of proceedings of another court. This term usually refers to an appellate court's examination of the proceedings and records of a lower court when a matter is being appealed. It is also used when a court wishes to reexamine an earlier decision.

Right: That which a person is legally entitled to have, do, or receive.

S

Sequester: To isolate; to separate. A jury is often sequestered from the public during a sensational trial.

Set aside: To annul, cancel, reverse, or void a judgment.

Sheriff: Chief law enforcement officer of a county.

Slander: To defame another's character, name, or reputation with false oral remarks.

Small claims court: A court characterized by informal proceedings that handles cases in which the amount in controversy is below an established maximum.

***Stare decisis* (the previous decision stands):** The practice of following judicial precedent. The principle that, since justice should be fixed, known, and applied equally to all, a decision made in one court should be followed by other courts in cases where the facts are substantially the same, unless the decision was made in error or was changed by a competent authority.

Statute: A law enacted by a legislature, either state or federal, that declares, commands, or prohibits something.

Statute of frauds: A law stipulating which contracts must be written to be enforceable in a court, such as a contract in which a third party agrees to the pay debts of another.

Statute of limitations: A law fixing the time period within which parties must begin litigation.

Statutory law: The category of law that is based on acts enacted by legislatures, as opposed to judge-made or common law.

Subpoena: A court order requiring the recipient to appear in a specified court at a specified time.

***Subpoena duces tecum* (under penalty you shall take with you):** A court order requiring the recipient to appear in a certain court at a certain time with the records, papers, documents, etc. specified in the subpoena.

Substantive law: The category of law that describes, defines, and regulates the rights and responsibilities of parties in legal relationships.

Suit: The legal procedure through which a party seeks a legal remedy for the alleged violation of a right, or seeks enforcement of a right.

Summons: A court order notifying the recipient that he/she is a defendant to a lawsuit and mandating the recipient's appearance in court at a certain time to defend himself/herself; failure to comply results in judgment against defendant.

Sustain: To support, approve, or maintain.

T

Testator: Male who dies leaving a will.

Testatrix: Female who dies leaving a will.

Testimony: Oral statement(s) made by a witness under oath, usually in connection with a legal proceeding.

Toll: To stop temporarily; to suspend or interrupt; for example, the statute of limitations is often tolled while the plaintiff is a minor.

Tort: A civil or private wrong resulting from the breach of a legal obligation (excluding breaches of contract) for which the court may provide a remedy.

Tort law: The branch of civil law that governs the redress of injuries suffered because of someone else's wrongdoing (excluding breaches of contract).

Tortfeasor: Wrongdoer; one who breaches a legal duty to another (excluding a breach of contract); one who commits a tort.

Trial: The phase of a lawsuit during which evidence, including testimony, is examined by a court for the purpose of settling disputed issues.

Trial court: Usually the first court to try a case; known as district courts in the federal court system; known as district, municipal, or superior courts in state systems.

Try: To examine evidence by judicial processes.

U

Undue influence: Indirectly or intangibly using one's power to sway another person so that person is unable to act freely, usually in the making of a will or a donation.

Unprofessional conduct: Behavior that violates or offends the standards of respectable members of the same profession, usually of an immoral, dishonorable, or illegal nature.

V

Vacate: To void or set aside, as in "to vacate a judgment."

Verdict: The finding or conclusion of the jury on issues of fact submitted to it for determination during a trial.

Vicarious liability: Indirect legal responsibility, such as the liability of an employer for certain wrongs committed by an employee while the employee was acting on the employer's behalf.

Vital statistics: A broad term referring to certain public records kept by a governmental agency upon statutory authority. Examples: birth, death, marriage, and divorce records.

Voir dire **(to speak the truth):** The term usually refers to examination of a prospective juror by the court and by the litigants' attorneys to determine the juror's impartiality and qualifications to try the case.

W

Waive: To relinquish voluntarily and intentionally a certain known right.

Warrant (an arrest): A written court order directing a law enforcement officer to arrest a certain person and bring him/her before a judicial officer.

Will: A document, prepared in accordance with certain legal requirements, that describes how a person wishes his/her property to be disposed of after his/her death.

Witness: A person who gives evidence to a court concerning matters of which he/she has firsthand knowledge.

> *Expert witness:* A person having superior knowledge of a subject about which he/she may testify; the knowledge is such that the ordinary person could not be expected to possess it, and is usually acquired by advanced study and specialized experience.

> *Hostile witness:* One whose relationship to the opposing party is such that his/her testimony may be prejudiced.

Wrongful death statute: A law that permits a deceased person's heirs to sue for losses when the death was caused by the negligence of another person.

Case Index

Index

Bloodborne pathogens, 185, 186
Board certified, 20, 21
Bobbit, Lorena, 141
Borrowed servant doctrine, 102, 103
Breach of confidence, 131, 132
Breach of contract as an intentional tort, 131, 132
  suits for, 114
    statutes of limitations in, 205
Broad consent form, use of, 71
Bureau of Narcotics and Dangerous Drugs (BNDD), 156

C

Cancer, as a reportable condition, 152
Canterbury Rule, 81
Captain of the Ship Doctrine, 100
Causes of litigation, 2-4, 211, 212
Caveat emptor, 67
Certificates, preparation of, 148,149
Certification, 20-22
  documentation of education and training, 21, 22
Chain of custody of specimens, 153
Chain of evidence, 153, 154
Character, defamation of, as intentional tort, 120, 121
Child abuse, 135-137
Churchill, Winston, 10
Civil law *(See Private law.)*
Civil Rights Act of 1964 (1991), 189, 190
Commercial law, 5
Common law, 8, 9

Communicable diseases, as a reportable condition, 151
Communication and care, as a prevention of conflict, 226, 227
Communications
  in the doctor–patient relationship, 45-50
    authorization to disclose information, 46-48
    confidentiality, legal basis of, 46
    faxing patient information, 48, 49
    privileged communication statutes, 50
    problems with confidentiality, 58-62
      HIV test results, 58, 59
      insurance companies, 59-61
      other, 61-62
  disclosure of patient's financial records, 202
Comparative negligence, doctrine of, 110, 111
Compensatory damages, 97
Complaint, 212, 213
Conception, as a bioethical issue, 245, 246
  artificial insemination, 245, 246
  frozen pre-embryos, 247
  in vitro fertilization and GIFT, 246
  surrogacy, 248
Confidentiality, in the doctor–patient relationship, 45-62
  disclosures, legally required, 50-57

by subpeona, 51
by statute to protect
    health or welfare,
    51, 52
to protect the welfare
    of the patient or
    third party, 52-54
guidelines for inexpe-
    rienced team mem-
    bers, 55-57
and members of the
    health care team,
    54, 55
of financial records, 202
Confidentiality problems, 58-
62
HIV test results, 58, 59
insurance companies, 59-
61
other, 61-62
Conflict, causes of, 211, 212
prevention of, 225-227
the facility: quality assur-
    ance/risk management,
    225
the individual: communi-
    cation and care, 226,
    227
resolution of, 212-224
alternatives for resolving
    disputes, 220-224
appeals phase, 220
litigation process, 212
pleadings phase, 212, 213
pretrial discovery phase,
    214-218
trial phase, 218-220
Congenital disorders, as a
reportable condition, 152
Consent
authority to, for, 63, 64
adults, 64
minors, 64-66

exceptions to necessity of,
    79
extending operations, 77-79
guidelines concerning, 74-
    76
HIV testing, 76, 77
in fiduciary relationships, 67
legal consequences, 79-81
    assault and battery, 79, 80
    negligence, 81
right to refuse, 67
Constitutional law, 4, 5
Consumer Protection Act
    (1969), 204
Consumer protection laws,
    201-209
financial philosophy and
    procedure, 202
professional courtesy, 202
confidentiality, 202
Equal Credit Opportunity
    Act of 1975, 203
Fair Credit Reporting Act
    of 1971, 203
Fair Debt Collections
    Practices Act of 1978,
    205, 206
charges to be avoided,
    203
statute of frauds, 204
small claims court, 206
    Federal Wage Garnish-
    ment Law (1970),
    206
liens in personal injury
    cases, 207
bankruptcy, 207
claims against estates, 208
Consequences, legal, of treating a patient without obtaining consent, 79-81
Contraceptives, need for
parental consent for provi-

115
Denial defense, 109
Depositions, 214
Discharge of doctor, by
     patient, 38
Disclosure of financial infor-
     mation, 202
Disclosures, legally required,
     50-57 *(See also Information
     disclosure.)*
Discovery rule, application of,
     for statutes of limitations,
     112
Discrimination and employ-
     ment, 187-198
   Age Discrimination in
       Employment Act
       (ADEA) of 1967
       (1974), 193
   Americans With Disabili-
       ties Act (ADA) (1990),
       193-196
   Civil Rights Act of 1964
       (1991), 189, 190
   Fair Labor Standards Act
       of 1939, 187, 188
   Family and Medical
       Leave Act of 1993, 196,
       197
   Immigration Reform and
       Control Act (1986) 198
   Sexual harassment, 190-
       192
   Social Security Act of
       1935 and the Employee
       Retirement Income
       Security Act
       (ERISA) of
       1974, 188
Doctor *(See also Physician.)*
   liability for employees, 101,
     102
   obligation for the standard

of care, 93
   obligations of in doctor–
       patient relationship, 31,
       32
   rights of in doctor–patient
       relationship, 30, 31
Doctor–patient contract, 25-33
Doctor–patient relationship
     *(See also Doctor–patient
     contract.)*
   communications in, 45-50
   confidentiality in, 45-62
   contracts in, 25-33
Domestic violence, 135-138
   Abuse of elderly and depen-
       dent adults, 137, 138
   Child abuse, 135-137
   Spousal abuse, 138
Drug addiction, need for
     parental consent for treat-
     ment of, 66
Drug Enforcement Admini-
     stration (DEA), 157
Drug usage *(See Controlled
     substances.)*
Duress, as intentional tort, 131

E
Elective sterilization, 253, 254
Emancipated minor, treatment
     of, 38, 39
Emergency care
   as exception to necessity of
       consent, 79
   and the Good Samaritan
       law, 39
   need for parental consent
       for minor, 64
Emotional distress, affliction
     of as an intentional tort,
     130, 131
Employee Retirement Income
     Security Act (ERISA) of

258-261
in doctor-patient relationship , 255, 256
Medical examiners, autopsies
and reports to, 146, 150
Medical-legal problems, contemporary, causes of, 2-4
Medical practice acts, 14, 15
prerequisites for licensure,
14
Medical records *(See Patient
health records.)*
Medical waste, 186, 187
Menendez brothers, 141
Mentally ill
commitment of, 154-156
Metabolic disorders, as a
reportable condition, 152
Minors
exceptions to consent for,
64-66
contraceptives, 66
court order, 65
drug addiction, 66
emancipated, 65
emergency treatment, 64
mature minor, 65
pregnancy, 66
sexually transmitted dis-
eases, 66
treatment of, 38, 39
Morris, R. Crawford, 3
Murder, as criminal offense,
133

N

Narcotics laws *(See Con-
trolled substances.)*
Negligence,
as an intentional tort, 86
as a legal consequence relating to consent, 80-82
as the proximate cause of

injury, 94
criminal, 134
and the law of agency, 100,
101
professional negligence
suits, 93-99
Nominal damages, 97
Nondoctor health care providers, medical ethics regarding referrals to, 239
Nonmedical personnel, medical ethics regarding referrals to, 239

O

Occupational health and safety, 184-186
bloodborne pathogens,
185, 187
medical waste, 186, 187
Occupational Safety and
Health Act, 184, 185
workers' compensation,
184
Occurrence rule, 112
Organ donation, medical
ethics regarding, 242
Organ transplantation, medical
ethics regarding, 242-244
anencephalic infants as
organ donors, 244
medical applications of
fetal tissue transplan-
tation, 244
Outrage, as intentional tort,
130, 131

P

Patient health records, 165-
177
contents, 168, 169
ownership, 169-171
purposes of, 166-168

as a legal document,
167
as an aid to communi-
cation, 166, 167
as an aid to practicing
medicine, 166
as basis of peer review,
168
for use in patient re-
search and training,
168
for use in professional
liability suits, 107-
109
record keeping guidelines,
172-175
release of information,
176-179
*subpoena duces
tecum*, 177-179
transfer of records,
176, 177
retention, 171
Patient representatives, medical ethics regarding referrals to, 239
Patient Self-determination
Acts, 259-260
Patient(s)
disclosures to protect welfare of, 52-54
ethics regarding doctor's
relationship with, 255,
256
famous patients, confidentiality in treating, 61, 62
invasion of privacy of, 125-
128
obligations of, in doctor–
patient relationship, 28-30
rights of, in doctor-patient
relationship, 27, 28
Pesticide poisoning, as a

reportable condition, 152
Pharmacists, liability of physician for negligence of, 103
Photographs of a patient, as an
invasion of privacy issue,
126, 127
Physician(s) *(See also Doctor.)*
medical ethics for, 234-262
in clinical situations, 240
in general practice, 234-
237
advertising, 235, 236
fees, 234, 235
medical records, 236,
237
in relationships with others, 238-240
doctors, 238, 239
nondoctor health care
providers, 239
nonmedical person-
nel, 239
media represen-
tatives, 239,
240
patient represen-
tatives, 239
in relationships with pa-
tients, 255, 256
costs of health care,
256
neglect of patient,
255
patient information,
255
unnecessary services,
256
obligation for the standard
of medical care, 86-92
Physician-patient contract *(See
Doctor–patient contract.)*
Physician-patient relationship
(See Doctor–patient rela-

Simpson, Nicole Brown, 138
Simpson, O.J., 138
Small claims court, 206
Social Security Act of 1935
and the Employee Retire-
ment Income Security Act
(ERISA) of 1974, 188,
Sources of law, 6-9
common, 8, 9
statutory law, 6, 8
Special damages, 98
Stare decisis, 8
Standard of medical care, 86-
92
Standard of care for allied
health professionals, 92
State courts, 11
Statutes *(See Public health
statutes and required
reports.)*
Statute of frauds, 27
Statute of limitations, 111-113
in breach of contract suits,
205
combination policy, 113
discovery rule, 112
last treatment rule, 112
occurrence rule, 112
time negligence rule, 112
Statutory law, 6, 8
Statutory offenses, 139
Sterilization, 252
Stillbirths, as a reportable condition, 148
Subpoena, disclosures
required by, 51
Subpoena duces tecum, 51
Substance and procedure, laws
of, 9-10
procedural, 9, 10
substantive, 9
Substantive law, 9
Surrogacy, 247

T

Technical defenses, 111-116
breach of contract suits, 114
interruption, 113
minors, 114
res judicata, 114, 115
statute of limitations,
111-113
Terminal illness
confidentiality problems, 61
ethics regarding, 259
patient self-determination
acts, 259, 260
Termination of doctor-patient
contract, reasons for, 33-38
abandonment, 34-36
discharge by patient, 38
withdrawal by physician,
36, 37
Testimonial statute, 50
Therapeutic sterilization, 253
Third party, information disclosures to protect welfare
of, 52-54
Time negligence rule, 112
Tort, intentional,
abortion fraud, 124
assault and battery, 118, 119
defamation of character,
120, 121
duress, 131
false imprisonment, 121,
122
fraud in the fiduciary relationship, 123, 124
insurance fraud, 124, 125
invasion of privacy, 125-128
malicious betrayal of professional secrets, 131, 132
tort of outrage, 130, 131
undue influence, 129, 130
Treatment, medical consent to,
63-84